Natural Remedies For

Horse Diseases

Mark Gilberd
Homoeopath. Medical Herbalist and Iridologist

Index

Herbal

Aniseed, Astragalus, Burdock, Celery Seed, Chamomile, Chaparral, Chaste Tree, Chickweed, Cleavers, Comfrey, Dandelion, Devils Claw, Dong Quai, Echinacea, Elder, Eyebright, Fennel, Fenugreek, Garlic, Ginger, Gingko Biloba, Ginseng Panax, Ginseng Siberian, Hops, Kelp, Lemon Balm, Licorice, Marshmallow, Meadowsweet, Mullein, Nettles, Parsley, Passion Flower, PauD'arco, Peppermint, Raspberry, Rose Hips, Sage, Slippery Elm Bark, Milk Thistle, Valerian, Wild Yam, Willow Bark, Wood Betony, Yellow Dock.

Homoeopathic Suppplement

Symptoms Guide

Disease Nosodes

Materia Medica

Aconite, Allium Cepa, Ant Tart, Apis, Arnica, Arsenic Album, Belladonna, Bellis Perinnis, Bryonia, Calendula, Cantharis, Carbo Vegetabilis, Causticum, Euphrasia, Hypericum, Ipecac, Kali Bich, Kali Carb, Lachesis, Ledum, Lycopodium, Nat Sulf, Nux Vom, Phosphorus, Pulsatilla, Rhus Tox, Ruta, Silica, Staphysagria, Symphytum, Tarantula Cuba, Urtica Urens.

Introduction
Welcome To The Animal Natural Remedy Series

These books are an effort to preserve the documentation of Natural Remedies used in the treatment of animals. In the past 100 years most of these treatments have been lost, especially in the treatment of cattle one of our most ancient of farm animals. Other reasons for writing these books is that I hate vet bills and people having to kill their farm animals or pets for economic reasons which I myself have been forced to do in the past on a Goat farm. Originally these books were put together as a field reference for myself for there is nothing worse than being in a paddock with a sick animal with the farmer, his hands on his hips waiting for you to perform and fix his animal.

Now the books have evolved and have had about 15 years of additions and are offered to you to teach you a new way of thinking. The books have evolved more by my different trainings. As a farmer I learnt to supplement the animals with the deficiencies of the soil so the books always start with the vitamins and minerals and their deficiency symptoms. As an Iridologist I tend to think and work with Body Systems such as The Nervous System or The Digestive System and concentrate on building them up with Nutrition and Herbs. As a Medical Herbalist I am trained to think holistically and design formulas that cover the whole being along with making the formulas easily absorbed. My Homoeopathic training teaches me to pay attention to the mind symptoms and to pay attention to what is really there not what I think is there and to treat and relieve the symptoms of the individual. Homoeopathy also shows how disease taints can be inherited and what to look for and how to treat them but best of all it gives me a special weapon to use when disaster strikes in the form of epidemics, these are called Disease Nosodes which are a preparation made from the disease product so you have a tool to help prevent the spread of disease. The books are set out in such a way as to teach you the correct use of Herbs e.g. thinking in body systems such as the Respiratory System or the Nervous System and in using herbs by their Medical Actions rather then that herb worked well last time. At the end of each system for example The Nervous System we have a section that gives you the common Actions used and needed for that section. Keeping with our example The Nervous System some of our Actions would be Anti-spasmodic, Sedative and Nervine Stimulants. After the explanation of the Action you have a list of herbs that are known to be strong in that action, this gives you more of a selection of herbs then what is mentioned in the text. Next we move on to the Homoeopathic Remedies for the condition which have the details to allow you to select a reasonably similar remedy. Homeopathy sits on a three legged stool. What this means is that if a remedy has at least three symptoms in the same strength as the symptoms you are trying to match then that remedy is a potential cure for your patient or if not cure it will offer the condition relief. The more symptoms you can match to the remedy the better the remedy will work for the rule is likes cure likes not vaguely similar cures. Homoeopathy (homo means same pathy means disease) is a good form of treatment for animals who usually respond to it fairly well and also it is very cheap to use and very easy to medicate unlike the herbs. A lot of effort has been put into the symptom details of the disease as it is very hard trying to diagnose when the animal can't answer your questions, so here you have to be very observant.

If used correctly this book makes you think and act more like a Professional Herbalist and broadens your view on what you are doing. With the Homoeopathics I have only really given you the leading remedies to put you on the right track, it would be worthwhile to invest in a good Materia Medica (Homoeopathic Remedy Reference) such as Boericke's which is one of the best for the Layman.

Main Reference Sources

The original base of the herbs I use were sourced from Juliette de Baïracli Levy's old Herbals, as hers are about the only Animal Herb References that have not been lost in time and they give you a lot of the old ancient herbs that have been used throughout most of history. To these I have added a lot of the more modern Herbs especially those that I use in my own work such as Astragalus and those that will soon be added after using for the first time on animals because there are just no substitutes. A good and recent example is Brahmi which I used in a cat recovering from a stroke because of my previous success in humans with this herb as it is supposed to rewire the brain around the damaged area and in its 3000 years of constant use someone must have used it on an Animal before. There are new herbs coming mainly from the Philippines, Indonesia, India and China but they are still being tried and tested and the average person wouldn't be able to get hold of them but the future looks far brighter than what it was 15 years ago when I started slowly putting this all together. We owe a lot to Juliette de Baïracli Levy for without her all these valuable herbs and how they were used would be lost. She has created a strong foundation that we can now build on.

Juliette de Baïracli Levy (11 November 1912 – 28 May 2009) was an English herbalist and author noted for her pioneering work in holistic veterinary medicine. Born to a wealthy Jewish family (her father was Turkish, her mother Egyptian) and raised in England with chauffeurs, maids, cooks, and gardeners. She knew as a child that she wanted to be a veterinarian. After studying veterinary medicine at the Universities of Manchester and Liverpool for two years she left England to study herbal medicine in Europe, Turkey, North Africa, Israel and Greece, living with gypsies, farmers and livestock breeders and recording their knowledge, especially the Gypsies. "I realized that if I wanted to learn the traditional ways of healing and caring for animals, I had to be where people still lived close to the land and close to their flocks," she says. "From Berbers, Bedouins, nomads, peasants, and gypsies in England, Israel, Greece, Turkey, Mexico, and Austria, I learned herbal knowledge and the simple laws of health and happiness. I never tired of traveling with my Afghan Hounds, always living with and learning from those around me." After living for some time on the Greek island Kythira she then resided in an old age home in Burgdorf, Switzerland leaving the world a better place.

For Homoeopathy my main hero is George Macleod not only for the success had based on his work but in my opinion he is a Homoeopathic Master up there with the greats and I admire his work in the use of Homoeopathic Disease Nosodes. All the high potencies mentioned are his work along with most of the Nosodes for as any trained Homoeopath knows and has had beaten into them during training you don't change the work of the masters. Unfortunately in our fast paced world not many people have time for Homoeopathy but I will say this, in the next Global Pandemic I and my family will be safe because I will make the Disease Nosode of it for I was trained by the Homoeopathic Masters.

George MacLeod (McLeod) (1912 – 1995) MRCVS DVSM Veterinary FF. Hom was a homeopathic vet, President of The British Association of Homeopathic Vets, Veterinary Consultant to The Homeopathic Development Foundation. George MacLeod was a graduate of Glasgow University and was one of the world's foremost authorities on Homeopathic treatment of animals. He was one of the few veterinary surgeons to use Homeopathic medicines wholly and exclusively. He was responsible for keeping Homeopathy available for animals in the UK, almost single-handedly, for the middle part of the 20th Century.

Other animal Homoeopaths sourced are Christopher Day, Edward Ruddock, and John Rush

Animal Natural Remedy Books

Natural Remedies For Cat Diseases
Natural Remedies For Dog Diseases
Natural Remedies For Goat Diseases
Natural Remedies For Sheep Diseases
Natural Remedies For Pig Diseases
Natural Remedies For Cow Diseases
Natural Remedies For Horse Diseases
Natural Remedies For Poultry Diseases

Mark Gilberd, Homoeopath, Iridologist, Medical Herbalist
Accredited With The Australian Traditional Medicine Society

Signs Of Ill Health In Your Horse

Horses that feel off color will generally appear listless. They may hang their heads and let their ears droop. They must feel something like we do when all we want to do is go to bed and sleep it off. You might find that they look tucked up with the tummy pulled in and they might even seem a little unsteady on their feet.

Physical Signs Of Ill Health
A Change In The Color Of Eye Membranes -
different colors can mean

Pale Membranes - might indicate anemia, chronic indigestion or worms.

Deep Red Membranes - are a sign of fever.

Deep Red Membranes with a Blue tinge - indicate pneumonia.

Yellow Membranes - might indicate a disorder of the liver.

Blue-Red Membranes - indicative of heart and circulatory problems.

A Change In Coat
If it is standing on end or staring and dull in appearance this is often a good indication of possible malnourishment. If you can pull a horses mane out easily this might also indicate ill health.

A Change In The Skin

Changes in the skin give several warning signs. Generally the skin of a horse in ill health will tighten up and does not rock freely back and forth as it should. The horse may be in the early stages of a general disease, or may have lice or be generally malnourished. Try the pinch test - does the skin spring back into place?

Signs Of Sweating

While excessive sweating may be caused by too much exercise if a horse is unfit, or by nervousness or excitement, the cause should be evident to you. If however the horse breaks out into a sudden cold sweat it might indicate acute physical pain or some form of mental unbalance. A uncharacteristic hot sweat is often a clear indication that your horse has a fever.

Puffy Or Swollen Limbs

Puffy limbs can denote various conditions of ill health. If the puffiness is due to a bone or joint problem your horse will obviously be lame. If the limbs are generally puffy all over the problem may be the heart or the lymphatic system. Localized puffiness may indicate a skin irritation or an injury

Temperature, Pulse And Respiration

You will often see TPR written in books on fitness and in articles in horse magazines. This refers to

Temperature, Pulse and Respiration. If your observations lead you to believe that your horse is off color check these 3 factors as they will either confirm or dispel your suspicions.

Temperature

A horse's normal temperature is 38 degrees C (100.5F). Any rise above this temperature indicates fever or some other problem and any drop in temperature is a sign of problems as well with shock being a good example here.

Taking The Pulse

Feel under the horses lower jaw (the bit that comes round in a semi-circle) until you come to the softness of a artery. This one is known as the maxillary artery and is usually the easiest from which to record the pulse. Gently move your fingers along the artery until you come to the place where it crosses the jawbone. Here you should be able to feel a definite beat. If a horse is generally fit and well the pulse rate at rest will be in the region of 35 to 40 beats per minute. If this rate exceeds 50 beats at rest you need to investigate further as the horse may be coming down with a fever or colic and may be in pain.

Taking The Respiration Rate

The respiration rate is the number of breaths (counting in plus out as one breath) per minute. This is simply checked by placing a hand over one of the horses nostrils and counting the breaths that you can feel within a minute or you can do it by watching and feeling the movement of the horses rib cage. While at rest the breaths should be even and regular and the respiration rate of a normal adult horse is between 8 and 12 breaths per minute, depending on the size of the horse - a Shire for example breathes at a lower rate (8) and a Shetland pony at a higher rate (12).

Minerals And Vitamins

If your animals live off your land and don't have any food or supplements brought in from outside then it is very important that you do a soil analysis and see if there are any deficiencies in your soil. This becomes even more important if you are having diseases and problems on a herd basis. What you need to do is find the deficiencies of your land and supplement your animals with the deficiencies until you manage to fix the problem. When you find the deficiencies of your land check the deficiency symptoms below and see if your stocks are showing any signs of them.

Calcium

Function - Assists in the contraction of muscles. Required for blood clotting. Assists in the production of hormones and enzymes. Works with phosphorus and Vitamin D to produce bone, bone is 35 percent calcium.

Sources - Green leafy forage, Limestone, Calcium Gluconate, Dicalcium Phosphate.

Herb Sources - Alfalfa, Blue Cohosh, Chamomile, Cleavers, Coltsfoot, Cayenne, Comfrey, Dandelion, Kelp, Mistletoe, Meadowsweet, Nettles, Parsley, Plantain, Raspberry, Rose Hips, Shepherds Purse, Yarrow, Yellow Dock.

Deficiencies - Rickets in young horses, Developmental Orthopaedic Disease, Azoturia, Poor muscle function, Impaired blood clotting, Joint problems and bone weakness.

Phosphorous

Function - Works with calcium for bone growth. Assists in energy metabolism. Makes up 15 percent of bone. Too much phosphorous will reduce the absorption of calcium during digestion.

Sources - Cereals, Dicalcium Phosphate.

Herb Sources - Alfalfa, Anise, Asparagus, Blue Cohosh, Caraway, Cayenne, Chickweed, Calamus, Dandelion, Dill, Fenugreek, Garlic, Golden Rod, Kelp, Liquorice, Linseed, Marigold, Meadowsweet, Parsley, Raspberry, Rose Hips, Sunflower, Yellow Dock.

Deficiencies - Overfeeding of phosphorous can lead to lameness, fragile bones, enlargement of the jaw bone, hyperparathyroidism

Magnesium

Function - Required for hemoglobin formation in the blood. Assists in bone formation. Assists in enzyme functions of the body.

Sources - Alfalfa, Clover, Bran, Linseed, Magnesium Carbonate.

Herb Sources - Alfalfa, Blue Cohosh, Broom, Carrot leaves, Cayenne, Dandelion, Hops, Marshmallow, Meadowsweet, Mistletoe, Mullein, Peppermint, Raspberry, Slippery Elm.

Deficiencies - Nervousness and excitability. Increased respiratory rates. Muscle tremors.

Aggressiveness and ill temper.

Sulphur

Function - Contains amino acids methionine and cystine. Assists in enzyme and hormone production.

Sources - Protein feeds and Green forage.

Herb Sources - Alfalfa, Burdock, Broom, Calamus, Coltsfoot, Cayenne, Daisy, Eyebright, Fennel, Garlic, Kelp, Marigold, Meadowsweet, Mullein, Nettle, Parsley, Plantain, Raspberry, Sage, Shepherds purse, Thyme, Yarrow.

Deficiencies - None recorded but overdosing can lead to loss of weight and appetite, colic, a yellow frothy discharge from the nose and labored breathing

Sodium Chloride

Function - Maintains the balance of fluids in the cells. Assists in muscle contractions. Removes waste products from the cells. Required in the production of bile. Maintains the health of the nervous system.

Sources - Salt and salt licks. Green forages especially Alfalfa.

Deficiencies - Dehydration, Poor Growth, muscle cramps. Over feeding of salt can result in high blood pressure.

Potassium

Function - Works with sodium to assist in correct

nerve function and muscular contractions. Assists in maintaining the correct fluid balance in the body.

Herb Sources - Alfalfa, Blue Cohosh, Borage, Carrot leaves, Chamomile, Coltsfoot, Comfrey, Couch Grass, Centaury, Dandelion, Elder, Eyebright, Fennel, Kelp, Ladies Mantle, Mistletoe, Meadowsweet, Mullein, Nettles, Parsley, Peppermint, Plantain, Raspberry, Shepherds Purse, Skullcap, Wormwood, Yarrow.

Source - Green forage and Molasses.

Deficiencies - Weight loss, Diarrhea, Muscle weakness.

Zinc

Function - Assists in the metabolism of nutrients. Required for the immune system to function correctly. Needed for healthy skin, hair and hooves. Assists in blood formation.

Sources - Yeast, Bran, Cereal Germ and Zinc Sulphate.

Herb Sources - Kelp and Marshmallow.

Deficiencies - Can lead to dry flaky skin, hair loss and poor growth loss.

Copper

Function - Essential in the formation of hemoglobin, cartilage and bone. Required for the correct utilization of iron in the body.

Sources - Grassland.

Herb Sources - Burdock, Chickweed, Chicory, Dandelion, Fennel, Garlic, Horseradish, Kelp, Parsley, Yarrow.

Deficiencies - Brittle weak bones, anemia, faded dull coat, in foals copper deficiency is associated with osteochondritis.

Manganese

Function - Required for the utilization of fats and carbohydrates. Essential for the formation of cartilage, assists in the formation of bones and enzymes.

Sources - Wheat Bran and Grasslands

Herb Sources - Kelp.

Deficiencies - Broodmares that become deficient can give birth to deformed foals whose bones are not correctly developed. Deficiency is fairly rare.

Iron

Function - Essential for the formation of hemoglobin and red blood cells.

Sources - Grasslands and Cereals.

Herb Sources - Alfalfa, Asparagus, Bilberry, Burdock, Blue Cohosh, Cayenne, Chicory, Comfrey, Dandelion, Gentian, Hawthorn, Hops, Mullein, Nettles, Parsley, Raspberry, Skullcap, Vervain, Yellow Dock.

Deficiencies - Anemia, Poor Performance, Poor growth in young stock.

Fluorine

Function - Essential for the formation of healthy teeth and bones, helps prevent tooth decay. Combines with calcium in the body and gives strength to the bones.

Sources - Pasture, Hay, Water and Limestone based supplements.

Herb Sources - Alfalfa, Beet leaves, Garlic, Water Cress.

Deficiencies - Deficiencies are rare but overdosing can occur especially where soils are rich in this mineral and the water has been treated with it as well. Signs of overdosing are discolored, mottled teeth, poor condition and rough coat and lameness in the joints.

Iodine

Function - Needed for correct functioning of the thyroid gland. Required for reproductive cycle to function correctly.

Sources - Kelp, Pasture and Mineral Licks

Herb Sources - Asparagus, Cleavers, Garlic, Kelp, Speedwell, Sarsaparilla.

Deficiencies - Abnormal oestrous cycle. Foals can be still born or born hairless while others may exhibit weakness and deformed joints. Overdosing can lead to enlarged thyroid glands.

Selenium

Function - Works with Vitamin E. Essential part of antioxidant enzymes which help which help to remove toxins from the system. A component of the amino acids Methionine and Cystine. Assists in maintaining a healthy immune system.

Sources - Pastures, Alfalfa, Brewers Grains and Linseed.

Deficiencies - In foals it can cause hair loss, dark urine, labored breathing and white muscle disease. Deficiencies in any horse can lead to azoturia. Overfeeding can cause poisoning.

Vitamins

Vitamin A (retinol)

Function - Needed for hormone synthesis, bone growth, and used in most of the mucous membranes of the body.

Sources - Carrots, Carotene in green leafy plants and Cod Liver Oil.

Herb Sources - Alfalfa, Burdock, Cayenne, Comfrey, Dandelion, Kelp, Marshmallow, Papaya, Parsley, Raspberry, Red Clover, Watercress, Yellow Dock.

Deficiencies - Night blindness, Excessive tears, Rough coat, Lack of appetite, Infections of the reproductive tract, Poor growth and weak bones and tendons.

B1 Thiamine

Function - Assists in metabolizing carbohydrates. Maintains a healthy nervous system. Assists in energy metabolism. Has been found to have a calming effect when feed to nervous horses. Can assist in the performance and stamina of competition horses. This vitamin is made by microflora in the intestines.

Sources - Good forage, Good hay, Cereal grains and Brewer's Yeast.

Herb Sources - Alfalfa, Burdock, Cayenne, Comfrey, Dandelion, Kelp, Marshmallow, Papaya, Parsley, Raspberry, Red Clover, Watercress, Yellow Dock.

Deficiencies - Weight loss, Muscular in coordination and missed heart beats. Deficiencies are fairly rare due to this vitamin being made in the intestines.

B2 Riboflavin

Function - Maintains a healthy nervous system. Assists in energy metabolism. This vitamin is also made in the intestines.

Sources - Green forage, Good hay and milk.

Herb Sources - Alfalfa, Burdock, Fenugreek, Kelp, Parsley, Watercress.

Deficiencies - Rough coat and dry skin, Conjunctivitis, Excessive tearing and may be connected with moon blindness. Deficiencies are fairly rare.

B3 Niacin

Function - Helps in the metabolism of nutrients and also with hormone and lipid syntheses. This vitamin is also made in the intestines.

Sources - Green forage especially Lucerne.

Herb Sources - Alfalfa, Burdock, Fenugreek, Kelp, Parsley, Sage.

Deficiencies - None recorded. Over dosing may cause dilation of blood vessels, sickness and itching of skin.

B5 Pantothenic Acid

Function - Assists in energy metabolism and the formation of anti-bodies.

Sources - Green forage, Cereals and Peas.

Deficiencies - Deficiency is rare as this vitamin is made in the intestines.

B6 Pyridoxine

Function - Assists in energy metabolism. Maintains health of the nervous system. Assists in the formation of hemoglobin in the blood. Maintains the health of the immune system. Heavily worked horses have benefited from B6 supplementation. This vitamin is made in the bowel.

Sources - Green forage and Cereal grains.

Herb Sources - Alfalfa, Chlorophyll.
Deficiencies - None recorded.

B12 Cyanocobalamin

Function - Assists in the production of red blood cells. Assists in energy metabolism. Fed to competition horses that are under stress. Can assist in putting on condition and correcting anemia. This vitamin is made in the bowel.

Sources - Green forages.

Herb Sources - Alfalfa, Chlorophyll, Dong Quai, Kelp.

Deficiencies - None recorded.

Biotin

Function - Assists in the metabolism of energy. Can assist in the improvement of poor quality hooves in some horses. Maintains sebaceous glands in the skin. Maintains bone marrow.

Sources - Yeast, Green forage and cereals.

Deficiencies - None recorded.

Choline

Function - Assists in the transport of fats stored in the liver to other areas of the body for use as energy. Maintains a healthy nervous system.

Sources - Natural Fats, Green leafy forage and Yeast cereals.

Deficiencies - Can lead to poor growth and increased storage of fats in the liver.

Folic Acid

Function - Assists cell metabolism. Required for red blood cell formation. Assists in general metabolism.

Sources - Green leafy forage

Deficiencies - None recorded in horses

Vitamin C (ascorbic acid)

Function - Essential for the formation of collagen tissue which is vital in tendons and cartilage. Essential for the utilization of essential amino acids lysine and proline.

Sources - Made in the liver and other body cells.

Herb Sources - Alfalfa, Burdock, Catnip, Cayenne, Chickweed, Dandelion, Hawthorn, Garlic, Horseradish, Kelp, Parsley, Plantain, Papaya, Raspberry, Rosehips, Shepherds Purse, Yellow Dock.

Deficiencies - None recorded. Supplementation has been given in periods of stress and growth.

Vitamin D

Function - Essential for the absorption of calcium and for growth maintenance and repair of bones and teeth.

Sources - Cut and dried plants, fish oils and through the skin after contact with sunlight.

Herb Sources - Alfalfa, Chlorophyll, Don Quai, Kelp.

Deficiencies - Reduced growth, weak bones and increased bone problems.

Vitamin E

Function - Helps with the immune system and is a powerful antioxidant. Helps stabilize cell membranes and acts on the reproductive system.

Sources - Leafy green forage, Good hay, Cereals and Alfalfa.

Herb Sources - Alfalfa, Dandelion, Dong Quai, Kelp, Raspberry, Rose Hips, Water Cress.

Deficiencies - Anemia, Swelling of joints, muscular in coordination and reduced stamina.

Vitamin K

Function - Helps in the clotting of blood and in calcium assimilation.

Sources - Made in the gut from green leafy forage.

Herb Sources - Alfalfa, Chlorophyll, Plantain, Shepherds Purse.

Deficiencies - Bleeding and longer blood clotting time.

The Digestive System

Acute Indigestion

Over eating or feeding on improper food is usually the cause for this condition along with maybe a change of diet.

Signs and Symptoms - These appear suddenly and include restlessness and signs of pain such as kicking at the abdomen. Frequent rolling may accompany a tympanitic abdomen along with rising and lying down at short intervals. Sweating and increased pulse rate occurs with discoloration of the conjunctiva. The symptoms may recede for a while and return just as bad a little time latter.

Herbal Treatment

Fennel is a good herb to use here 2 handfuls of the whole plant feed raw twice daily and give the seeds as well for they are the main cure for indigestion maybe a hand full a day. I would give half a handful as soon as I noticed the problem and the rest about 45 minutes latter for by this time I would of expected to see some improvement. Another good herb for this condition is aniseed which is especially good for young animals again the average dose is one heaped handful of seeds a day. These two herbs have very high essential oil components (aromatic) and it is the action from this that we are using to help the problem. The action is called Carminative. Other herbs to consider are Peppermint, Ginger and Chamomile.

Homoeopathic Treatment

Nux Vomica 6C - Especially if the condition arises from indigestion of indigestible fodder, constipation is usually present. Dose every 2 hours for 4 doses.

Colchicum 6C - Tympanic abdomen, animal passes flatus frequently, Dose every 2 hours for 3 doses.

Colocynthis 6C - Animal rolls in acute pain with head turns towards flanks. Dose every 2 hours for 4 doses.

Arsenicum Alb 1M - Animal restless, worse towards midnight, thirsty for small quantities of water, skin dry and scruffy. Dose every hour for 3 doses.

Lobelia 6C - Salivation and profuse sweating, appetite often remains good, flatulence often occurs. Dose 4 times daily for one day.

Lycopodium 6C - Accompanying liver symptoms such as yellowish discoloration of the conjunctiva and tenderness over the liver region, highly fermentable foods aggravate. Dose every 2 hours for 4 doses.

Carbo Veg 6C - Abdomen tense due to flatulence with comatose symptoms, flatus very offensive, symptoms worse lying down. Dose every hour for four doses.

Colic

There can be many causes for this common disorder some of the usual ones are eating frost encrusted grass and heavy feeding when the animal is exhausted after a hard day's work. Another cause is indigestible foods such as moldy, damp or fermenting hay, very new hay, too much clover and over feeding with beans and peas.

This condition is referred to as spasmodic or flatulent according to the symptoms arising. Spasmodic colic implies a cramping or spasm of the intestine. Animals of a excitable temperament are more disposed to the condition than those of a more lethargic nature.

Flatulent colic as the name implies is accompanied by excessive formation of flatus. In each type the pulse becomes thready and the conjunctiva discolored.

Signs and Symptoms - Initially there is restlessness, pawing the ground and kicking at the abdomen. The animal lies down and may roll around violently or it may lie flat, occasionally looking around at the flank. The spasms pass off but return after a short interval. The expression is anxious and the respirations are increased. With flatulent colic there are the additional symptoms of tympany and tense abdomen. There are rumbling noises from the bowel and frequent passing of wind. We can distinguish colic from other problems by the fact that the pains come and go at intervals and that the animal does not lose its strength very quickly.

Herbal Treatment

Read the herbal section above - Indigestion - because the two herbs mentioned there aniseed and fennel can be helpful in the treatment of colic. If the pains of colic are not speedily and effectively relieved death can result in many cases. Preventative treatment is important because once a horse is attacked by colic then it is most likely that it will happen again in the future. A useful preventative for flatulent horses who you may think are getting into trouble is a handful of charcoal tablets as these tablets will absorb a lot of the toxins and gas and could prevent the problem going further. This is a old recipe for colic I will quote it as it is written. (Where the Gentian and Licorice are mentioned we could use the tinctures instead.) For the relief of the actual pains give a drench as follows - into a quart of warm milk stir 1 tablespoon of grated gentian root, one tablespoon of melted Spanish licorice juice, half a teaspoonful of Oil of Peppermint, four tablespoons of melted honey. If the drench does not give quick relief than half a desert spoonful of powdered ginger should be added to the mixture. Other herbs to consider for this condition are Peppermint, Chamomile, Lemon Balm and for the pain think of giving Wild Yam. In the Homoeopathics below think of Colocynth 1M for the pain. For this condition Pat Coleby gives a drench of 4 tablespoons of Vitamin C powder (sodium ascorbate) immediately along with 25cc by injection into the muscle on each side of the neck.

Homoeopathic Treatment

Aconite 6C - Always in the early stages, one dose every hour for 4 doses

Belladonna 1M - Full bounding pulse early in the condition, sweating, dilated pupils and excitability, skin hot and smooth. Dose every 2 hours for 4 doses.

Colchicum 6C - Distension of abdomen and rumbling of flatus, lower parts of the bowel become distended and can be felt on the right side, animal tends to remain standing. Dose every hour for 3 doses.

Colocynth 1M - When spasmodic colic has severe pain and appears to result from having eaten green food. Motions are watery with wind. Dose every 4 hours for 4 doses.

Nux Vom 6C - If the attack was brought on by eating indigestible food or overeating. Straining to pass dung or urine, animal lies on its side looking uneasy, bending head towards flank. Dose every 2 hours for 4 doses.

Note - In extremely acute cases administer the doses every 10 to 15 minutes. Generally 5 or 6 doses should be sufficient followed by the extended times given above.

Inflammation Of The Bowels

The symptoms of this disease are very like those of colic only in the latter disease there are intervals of rest or cessation of pain and there is little or no alteration of the pulse but in inflammation of the bowels there is no abatement of pain but here the animal is continually lying down and rolling about getting up then dropping down suddenly. The pulse is very much quickened, small and hard, the artery appears like a cord under the finger, the extremities are cold, the animal frequently turns his head towards the flanks, the abdomen is hard and tender and as the disease advances the breathing becomes accelerated. The eyes become staring and wild, a cold sweat breaks out all over the body, this state continues for some time when suddenly the animal appears to get better, he gets up and stands quietly, the eyes loose there luster, the extremities become deadly cold and there is tremulous agitation of the muscles particularly the fore part of the body, after a short time he begins to stagger and totter about and soon falls down head long and dies. This description is probably over a hundred years old and is fairly dramatic and is a close copy of the original written by a Doctor John Rush.

Herbal Treatment

Here could be the time to call a vet. The treatment is similar to colic especially at first. Spanish Gypsies use a brew of the herb called horsetail for soothing the inflamed bowels. Hops is the specific for irritable bowel especially for those of a nervous nature it also has an antiseptic action which may be of use in this condition. Think of the anti-inflammatory herbs especially Meadowsweet and Wild Yam which would also help with the pain. Another herb to think of is Peppermint for its pain and antiseptic actions. Another action that may prove useful here is that of the Demulcents which coat and sooth inflamed areas, two good and safe ones to use are Comfrey and Marshmallow.

Homoeopathic Treatment - as stated by Doctor Rush

Aconite 6C - Is the chief remedy to depend upon in this disease and should be repeated frequently till a calm is established which generally takes place in one hour. Dose is 6 drops every ten minutes.

Arsinic Alb 6C - If after the use of Aconite and some symptoms still remain, especially if the disease has been produced by green food or by drinking cold water when heated. Dose 6 drops at half hour intervals or longer if symptoms recede.

Rhus Tox 6C - If the extremities are alternately hot and cold with sweating of the belly and a frequent discharge of urine. Dose same as Arsenic Alb.

Colocynthis 6C - If Arsenic does not remove all the symptoms, especially if it is accompanied with colic and there are bloody evacuations. Dose 6 drops every half or one hour.

Cantharis 6C - If there is retention of urine.

Diarrhea

Transient, self-limiting diarrhea may result from sudden changes in diet, excitement, temperature or transport and provided that faecal consistency returns to normal within 2 to 3 days is of little consequence. Usually once the offending material has passed through the intestines the problem will cease. Diarrhea may be a accompaniment of disease or It can also happen at the beginning of spring as the new growth arises.

Signs and Symptoms - Frequently there is straining when passing evacuations and shreds of mucous membrane may be seen. Motions may be watery or mucoid, sometimes slimy varying in color according to the underlying cause. The stool may be passed with difficulty shown by straining or it may come easy. Superpurgation may arise from the over use of purgatives or by giving a to larger dose, it may also be seen towards the end of febrile (fever) diseases as a result of a disordered metabolism e.g. liver dysfunction. Signs can be passage of flatus accompanied by signs of abdominal uneasiness e.g. looking round at flanks. If too much fluid is lost the legs may get cold and the body temperature may fall. In very severe cases a vet must be called because sometimes the ability to absorb fluids from the gut can be lost so the fluids have to be replaced via the blood and often require tens of liters of fluid. Chronic diarrhea is usually caused by worms especially if it gets worse in summer and the horse had been in a poor condition throughout winter.

Herbal Treatment

This should begin with a laxative drench to sweep out the putrid matter from the intestines. A quick and effective drench is one to two full ounces of Epsom's Salts dissolved in half a pint brew of Dill seed water or Senna pods. One small handful of Dill seeds boiled for 5 minutes in one pint of water and brewed for 2 hours (cover while brewing so as to keep the essential oils in). Fast the horse for 24 hours following the drench and then give a Garlic brew or Garlic capsules for internal disinfecting in the evening. Introduce the animal back to its normal diet slowly and gently while observing the effects. Highly recommended in all forms of diarrhea is to thicken the molasses feed with powdered Slippery Elm Bark. This herbal substance acts as an internal poultice. It does not falsely cure the diarrhea by blocking the bowel as with chalky chemical powder products, it cures in the true sense of the word by its soothing and healing powers. Slippery Elm in the gruel has saved the life of many a young animal. Slippery Elm is one of the main herbs to think of in diarrhea especially for the very young. The herb is mainly used as a demulcent to sooth inflamed intestines but this herb also has a mild astringent action which is probably enhanced by the coating demulcent action bringing it in close contact with the intestinal wall. This herb is also a nutritive herb in its own right and when it is mixed with raw honey and fed to the very young in very bad health it can actually keep them alive for far longer than normal; the raw honey would also have a antibacterial action. In general it is the Astringent herbs that are used in stopping diarrhea and especially Dysentery as the astringent action contracts the pores in the intestines restricting the flow of liquid inside. Cranesbill, Raspberry and Shepherds Purse are strong astringents though Meadowsweet would be good to add to them because of its other actions.

Homoeopathic Treatment

Aconite 30C - Give at the onset of the problem especially if it arises from cold or there is fever.

Mercurius Cor 200C - Motions are slimy and may contain a little blood, the condition is often worse during the night and the horse salivates a lot. Dose every 2 hours for 4 doses.

Arsenic Alb 1M - Motions pale, watery and excoriate the skin around the anus, signs of abdominal pain, thirst for small quantities of water, worse after midnight, there is restlessness and weakness. Odor from stools is carrion like. Dose every 2 hours for 4 doses.

Byronia 6C - Condition brought on by cold dry winds or sudden change of temperature or by drinking large quantities of cold water. Dose 3 times daily for 3 days.

Nux Vom 6C - Overeating or partaking of indigestible food, diarrhea may be preceded by attacks of colic.

Dulcamara 200C - Attacks of diarrhea follow exposure to damp, stools are green and slimy, more prevalent in summer after sudden fall in temperature. Dose every 2 hours for 4 doses.

Colocynth 6C - Attack is accompanied by severe abdominal pain, animal lies down and rises frequently, bending neck towards abdomen, food and drink produces jelly like slimy stools. Dose every half hour for 4 doses followed by one dose every 4 hours.

China 30C - Weakness due to loss of body fluid. This remedy is especially useful in chronic cases. Dose 3 times daily for 3 days.

Podophyllum 6C - Long standing cases, stools watery and fetid attacks worse in the morning, there may be prolapse of rectum, very useful in young animals. Dose 3 times daily for 3 days.

Constipation

This condition accompanies many diseases but may arise independently as a result of bad management or may even be caused from lack of sufficient fluid intake.

Signs and Symptoms - Severe straining and passage of small hard lumps of dung which may be covered with slimy mucous, spots of blood may be present on the lumps and in severe cases febrile signs may appear such as reddened conjunctiva and quickened pulse.

Herbal Treatment

Look to the diet so as to try and find and correct the cause as constipation is more common in stall kept animals. Sometimes warm water enemas can be used if there is a obstruction of dry dung. A purge that was much used by old fashioned herbalists was 2 tablespoons of powdered licorice, 1 desert spoonful of powdered ginger, made into a paste in two ounces of castor oil and rolled into balls for dosing. A non-oil purge is the Senna purge. For the Senna purge a horse can take 20 or more large pods soaked in half a pint of water with a quarter of a teaspoon full of ginger powder added. Laxatives are the main action we commonly associate with constipation but there is another two to consider with the first being Aperient which is an action name for a mild laxative and the other being Cholagogues which stimulates the release of bile from the gallbladder which can relieve gallbladder problems, but in this case bile is also the body's natural laxative so Cholagogues have a laxative effect as well as a effect on the liver.

Homoeopathic Treatment

Nux Vom 6C - Uncomplicated cases, when there is ingestion of indigestible food. Dose every 2 hours for 3 doses in mild cases. In animals subject to a more chronic condition give a 1M dose night and morning for 2 days.

Sulphur 6C - Abdomen sensitive to pressure and colicky symptoms after drinking. This remedy can most usefully be employed in conjunction with Nux Vom giving the remedies in alternation.

Hydrastis 30C - General catarrhal states, signs of stiffness over lumber region, liver dysfunction and jaundice may be present. Dose 3 times daily for 3 days.

Mag Mur 6C - Liver dysfunction, yellow tongue and other signs of jaundice may appear, stools small and crumbly, Dose 3 times daily for 3 days.

Bryonia 6C - Stools large hard and may contain blood especially in young animals. Dose 3 times daily for 3 days.

Liver Problems

Jaundice

This occurs as a symptom of inflammation of the liver. Sluggish function without inflammation may also produce jaundice. It is also sometimes associated with pneumonia. Obstruction of the bile ducts is an obvious cause. The main cause may be a unsuitable diet especially over prolonged use of concentrated unnatural cakes and meals. Also vermifuges (wormers) may over time damage the liver and produce jaundice.

Signs and Symptoms - The mucous membranes of the eye, mouth and nose become tinged with yellow and the skin also shows this discoloration. Urine becomes dark green because of the presence of bile, constipation may be present, faeces is light in color and in some cases there may be edema of the limbs.

Herbal Treatment

It is the derangement of the bile flow which is the basic cause for this complaint and until it is normalized the yellow pigment will continue to noticeable especially in the eyes. Give a short fast with a non-oily purge (senna pods - see constipation). All fatty foods should be avoided in the diet also avoid giving pulse foods. Give a abundance of Dandelion in the diet the roots can be grated and included as well. Also recommended are Cleavers and Centaury. Otherwise the diet should be mainly grass and other leafy green vegetables, bran, molasses, carrots and seaweed.

The horse can also respond well to a brew of Hops for the relief of jaundice. Speedwell herb 3 handfuls a day is a popular remedy of French Gypsies. The main herbal actions to think of here are those of the Chologogues. Another herb worthy of serious consideration is Milk Thistle, always think of this herb for serious liver problems.

Speedwell - Used for jaundice, impure blood, dysentery, gastric insufficiency, coughs asthma etc.

Homoeopathic treatment

Aconite 30C - Give at the onset of the problem especially if it arises from cold or there is fever.

Berberis Vulgaris 30C - Sluggish liver conditions with tenderness over lumber region. Skin yellowish, urinary symptoms present. Dose 3 times daily for 3 days.

Chelidonium 6C - Pain and tenderness over right shoulder area. Strong yellow discoloration of visible mucous membranes. Obstruction of bile ducts. Dose 3 times daily for 3 days.

China 30C - Weakness and debility, abdominal pain, stools yellow and fluid, increasing weakness. Dose every 3 hours for 4 doses.

Lycopodium 200C - Flatulent state, indifferent appetite, abdominal tympany after eating, mucous membranes grayish yellow and urine loaded with red sediment, Dose night and morning for 5 days.

Mag Mur 30C - Enlargement of liver with difficulty in urination, jaundice and abdominal pain pronounced. Dose night and morning for 4 days.

Hepatitis

Inflammation of the liver may be caused by a number of varying substances, some in the horse being viral or other infectious agents. This condition can be acute or chronic.

Signs and Symptoms - In the acute form the animal is dull and disinclined to move, muscular weakness and anorexia are common signs and there may be nervous excitability. Urine is scanty and highly colored. The faeces are clay colored and soft after initial constipation in the early anorexia stage. Yawning and lethargy are seen and there may be a tendency to fall forward or press the head against a wall or any convenient object. There is conjunctival discoloration and the mucous membranes of the mouth and nose are yellow and furred looking. Pain over the right scapula area produces slight lameness and is also evident on palpitation of the liver area. Photosensitization may occur in animals which are exposed to sunlight and feed on green food. Chronic states may show edema and jaundice more commonly then in the acute form.

Herbal Treatment

See also jaundice. The best herb for hepatitis is Milk Thistle which is also known as St Marys Thistle. This is best given alone at the beginning of the crisis until the worst is over.

Homoeopathic Treatment

Phosphorus 200C - Acute form, stools whitish either soft or hard, jaundice and purpura like hemorrhages occur, urine is muddy looking, pain in abdomen. Dose 3 times daily for 3 days.

Bryonia 6C - Better at rest, relief from pressure over liver, dry coughing may accompany the condition, stools hard dark dry, urine scanty and hot. Dose 3 times daily for 3 days.

Chelidonium 6C - Pain and tenderness over right shoulder area. Strong yellow discoloration of visible mucous membranes. Obstruction of bile ducts, acute stage, Dose 3 times daily for 3 days.

Hepar Sulph 200C - Suspected hepatic abscess shown by presence of purulent urine which has a greasy look, suppurative involvement may be evident elsewhere e.g purulent rhinitis. Dose night and morning for 5 days.

Lycopodium 200C - More chronic form in the early stages of cirrhosis, ascites usually present (edema of abdomen). Urine contains reddish sediment and is passed copiously during the night. Dose night and morning for 2 weeks.

Herbal Overview Of The Digestive System

In dealing with problems of the digestive system it's always best to start with a purge so as to clean the system and bowels out. This is very important especially when you do not know what you are dealing with because you are purging out hopefully most of the toxins that are causing the condition. After the purge isolate and fast the animal for 24 hours and see what happens. When you are unsure on what is going on and it seems serious especially when the temperature is rising start on the Garlic and Echinacea straight away as the Echinacea is also used to treat septicemia and to attack blood borne toxins along with being a immune booster and with Garlic being antiviral and antibacterial we have together a good strong initial attack. If you look at the herbal treatment sections above you will see they cover most of the conditions of the digestive system and should give you helpful information.

Below are a list of Herbal Actions that are used for the digestive system read through them and become familiar with them for in Herbal Medicine you always think in actions needed not the Herb needed this way the mind stays on the big picture.

Herbal Actions For The Digestive System

Anti-biotic - Always start with Garlic as this is both anti-bacterial and anti-viral as well as being used for killing parasites and worms, your initial attack begins here.

Herbs - Echinacea, Garlic, Myrrh, Pau D' Arco.

Anti-emetic - Can reduce a feeling of nausea and can help to relieve or prevent vomiting.

Herbs - Cayenne, Fennel, Meadowsweet, Peppermint.

Anti-inflammatory - Helps the body to combat inflammations, there will always be pain, heat and maybe fever when these are called for. Herbs mentioned under demulcents will often act in this way especially when they are applied to coat for example an inflamed intestine or any other inflamed organ.(Slippery Elm).

Herbs - Cranesbill, Chamomile, Feverfew, Ginger, Golden Rod, Ladys Mantle, Liquorice, Marshmallow, Meadowsweet, Marigold, Pau D' Arco, Witch Hazel, Wormwood.

Anti-microbial - Helps the body destroy or resist pathogenic micro-organisms.

Herbs - Aniseed, Cayenne, Echinacea, Garlic, Gentian, Marigold, Myrrh, Peppermint, Rosemary, Rue, Sage, Thyme, Wormwood.

Antispasmodic - Prevents or eases spasms and cramps especially of the intestines.

Herbs - Aniseed, Angelica, Chamomile, Fennel, Rosemary, Rue, Sage, Skullcap, Thyme, Valerian, Vervain.

Anti-viral - Astragalus, Cats claw, Echinacea, Garlic, Myrrh?, Pau D'Arco.

Anthelmintic - Destroys or expels worms from the digestive system.

Herbs - Garlic, Tansy, Wormwood, Thyme, Rue.

Aperient - Mild laxative.

Herbs - Burdock, Dandelion.

Astringent - Contracts tissue which in turn reduces discharges, these herbs contain tannins. In the digestive system they can be used to stop diarrhea and in the treatment of ulcers. Most astringents also

have a anti-bacterial action.

Herbs - Agrimony, Bear Berry, Cranesbill, Comfrey, Eyebright, Golden Rod, Hops, Ladys Mantle, Marigold, Marshmallow, Meadowsweet, Nettles, Raspberry, Sage, Rosemary, Slippery Elm, Shepherds Purse, St Johns Wort, Slippery Elm, Thyme, Witch Hazel, Yarrow.

Bitters - Herbs that taste bitter act as stimulating tonics for the digestive system.

Herbs -Burdock, Feverfew, Gentian, Hops, Horehound, Rue, Tansy, Wormwood.

Carminative - Stimulates peristalsis of the digestive system and relaxes the stomach and helps remove gas and wind from the system. These herbs are usually rich in volatile oils.

Herbs - Aniseed, Angelica, Cayenne, Chamomile, Fennel, Garlic, Ginger, Golden Rod, Hyssop, Horseradish, Juniper, Parsley, Peppermint, Penny Royal, Sage, Rosemary, Tansy, Thyme, Valerian, Wormwood.

Cholagogue - Stimulates the release of bile from the gallbladder which can relieve gallbladder problems, bile is also the body's natural laxative so cholagogues have a laxative effect as well.

Herbs - Agrimony, Blue Flag, Dandelion, Fumitory, Gentian, Marigold, Milk Thistle, Yellow Dock.

Demulcent - Soothes and protects irritated or inflamed internal tissues.

Herbs - Bear Berry, Corn Silk, Coltsfoot, Comfrey, Fenugreek, Liquorice, Marshmallow, Milk Thistle, Mullein, Oats, Plantain, Slippery Elm.

Diaphoretic - Aids the skin in the elimination of toxins and produces sweat thus reducing the temperature of fevers.

Herbs - Angelica, Black Cohosh, Cayenne, Chamomile, Elder, Elecampane, Fennel, Garlic, Ginger, Golden Rod, Guaiacum, Hyssop, Lime Blossom, Peppermint, Sarsaparilla, Thyme, Vervain, Yarrow.

Hepatic - Tones and strengthens the liver, may increase the flow of bile.

Herbs - Agrimony, Blue Flag, Dandelion, Fennel, Fumitory, Gentian, Horseradish, Hyssop, Motherwort, Milk Thistle, Vervain, Wormwood, Yarrow.

Laxative - Promotes the evacuation of the bowels.

Herbs - Burdock, Dandelion., Fumitory, Horseradish, Licorice, Senna

Parasiticide - Kills parasites and insects.

Herbs - Aniseed, Rosemary,

Sialagogue - Stimulates the secretion of saliva.

Herbs - Blue flag, Cayenne, Gentian, Ginger.

The Respiratory System

Sinusitis

Catarrhal conditions of the upper respiratory tract may involve the sinuses leading to a chronic sinusitis. This condition can also be caused by dental problems, one clue you will get if it is a tooth abscess is that the discharge will smell foul so make sure this is not the cause.

Signs and Symptoms - There is a discharge of pus from the nostrils with swelling over the nasal bones and maxillary region. Dullness on percussion is herd over the affected area. Lungs and chest sound clear.

Herbal Treatment

Juliette de Bairacli Levy treats this condition by fasting and internal cleansing (see common colds) along with heavy dosing with garlic. Rinsing out the nostrils with 1 teaspoon of fresh lemon juice to a cup of tepid water. To my way of thinking Ginger and all the hot herbs are worth considering because they thin mucous which is getting to the point of the problem as you can't get thick mucus out of a small hole and they are very small in the sinus cavities. What usually happens is the trapped mucous increases leading to the bone aching pains of this condition which leads us to our next herb Wood Betony which is used for pains in the head and face. For this condition in its chronic state the herb to use is Fenugreek as this not only thins the mucous but it is also a lymphatic cleanser so it will start to slowly move all the rubbish out. The golden rule here is that for every year the condition has existed you will need at least one month of treatment. For the acute condition think of Garlic, Echinacea, Golden Rod, Eyebright if the eyes are affected. Actions to consider for this condition are Anti biotic, Anti catarrhal, Anti-inflammatory and if you believe that the mucus is burning or irritating the skin consider the Action of Demulcents and Emollients. I would also give a good dose of Vitamin C till the situation improves to help boost the immune system.

Homoeopathic Treatment

Hepar Sulph 2OOC - Sensitivity to draughts and cold, extreme sensitivity to touch or pressure on the affected area. Dose night and morning for one week.

Hydrastis 30C - Pus bland flowing freely from nostrils. Dose 3 times daily for 6 days

Kali Bich 200C - Long standing cases showing tough stringy discharge. Dose night and morning for 5 days.

Silica 200C - Chronic cases showing thin whitish pus associated with affections of the maxillary and nasal bones. Dose night and morning for 5 days.

Arsenic Alb 1M - Discharge acrid tending to burn the nostrils, restless, worse after midnight. Dose once daily for 5 days.

Cough

While coughing is frequently associated with various pulmonary infections it may arise as a seemingly independent syndrome and takes various forms.

1. Pleuritic cough - Short and dry and the animal shows pain while coughing.
2. Bronchitic cough - Starts dry and frequent, becomes moist and soft.
3. Simple catarrhal cough - Usually moist and infrequent.
4. Pneumonic Cough - Frequent, may contain rust colored fibrinous deposits in the sputum.
5. Stomach or intestinal cough - Various forms dependent on alimentary disorders.

Herbal Treatment

This is often present in wormy horses and in animals long confined in the dusty and vitality impairing atmosphere of stables. I have decided to write the treatment section exactly as it was done in the past and in brackets give you the tinctures used today. For the local relief of the cough give a drench of brewed cherry twigs (Wild Cherry Bark Tincture), one pint, with one table spoon of honey and one table spoon of black treacle added. An alternative and proved excellent drench is a brew of equal parts Pine Needles and Elder twigs, blossoms or leaves (Elder Tincture), 2 handfuls of each of the herbs brewed in a quart of water. Give a drench of one pint. Coltsfoot can replace the Pine or Elder. When mouths are sore or inflamed bath with a brew of Sage. The following Farrier recipe makes a excellent cough drop for horses - Anise seeds one pound, ground ginger one pound, ground licorice one pound and one handful of caraway seeds. Add sufficient treacle to form a mass and roll into balls. Give one ounce of this mixture every morning and fast the horse for about an hour allowing it time to work. Now let's take a more modern approach. Always try to find the cause for this will usually determine the Actions you will need. The main needed Action here is that of the Expectorants with the best being Horehound and Coltsfoot especially when you don't know the cause as these are good all round herbs for the respiratory system and can treat most conditions mentioned in this chapter just by themselves. Wild Cherry Bark mentioned above has a sedative action on the main nerve of the lungs and is used more for the spasmodic whooping type of cough. Other actions to consider are Anti-Inflammatories especially where there is obvious pain on coughing or the cough is hoarse sounding along with this action always consider the Demulcents so they can sooth the raw area and relieve the pain. An example of a herb that has all three of these actions is Mullein and also Coltsfoot. If there is lots of mucous coming up have a good look at the Anti-Catarrhal herbs and try to find one that covers a lot of the other actions you need. If the coughing is from worms consider the Anthelmintic herbs.

Homoeopathic Treatment

Bryonia 6C - Pleuritic cough, dry, symptoms worse on movement, better from pressure or pressure over the affected area. Dose 3 times daily for 3 days.

Belladonna 30C - cough accompanied by full pulse,

dry cough, hot smooth skin, dilated pupils, nervous symptoms. Dose every 2 hours for 4 doses.

Drosera 6C - Spasmodic coughs of a chronic nature, sometimes associated with asthmatic symptoms worse at night when the animal lies down. Dose every 2 hours for 4 doses.

Nux Vom 6C - Origin in digestive upsets, dry cough, hoarse, spasmodic worse in the morning. Dose 3 times daily for 3 days.

Causticum 30C - Cough relieved by drinking, expectorations scanty. Dose night and morning for 4 days.

Arsenic Alb 1M - Cough worse after midnight, animal restless, thirsty with dry skin, cough worse after drinking even small quantities. Dose night and morning for 4 days.

Spongia 30C - Cough worse on inspiration and worse towards midnight, relieved by drinking, sometimes associated with heart disease. Dose night and morning for 3 days.

Sticta 6C - Cough originates more in trachea, is worse in the evening and during the night and on inspiration. Dose 3 times daily for 3 days.

Coryza - Common Cold

Inflammation of the nasal mucous membranes may arise from exposure to cold and damp and frequently attacks horses that are in poor condition or badly housed. Coryza (running mucous) has a tendency to extend to the laryngeal and lower respiratory area leading to a possible bronchitis or pneumonia.

Signs and Symptoms - Early signs include sneezing and swelling of the eyelids, followed by a thin mucous discharge from the nose. Discharge soon becomes thick and catarrhal; the horse goes off its food and may have a great thirst, staring coat, drooping head mane and tail. Most cases resolve quickly but a chronic form may supervene in poorly nourished animals. Laryngitis and cough may accompany the condition the former being associated with throat swelling.

Herbal Treatment

Fast for one or two days, this should then be followed by a cleansing diet which should include abundant carrots (Vitamin A for the lungs),also add a teaspoonful of Paprika to the food. Avoid for some weeks all the nitrogenous foods such as peas and beans and also avoid oats. Dusty hay must be rigidly excluded from the diet all hay given during the treatment should be well dampened with a solution of water and molasses. Dose with Garlic night and morning and if the throat seems to be sore then give twice daily a drench of honey and elder blossom with sage brew. Honey and lemon juice (Vitamin C) is also excellent for this press the juice of 2 large ripe lemons into half a pint of warm water and stir in 2 tablespoons of honey. The discharging nostrils should be cleansed with a brew of Elder Blossom and Meadowsweet on cotton wool, diluted lemon juice can also be used. The only addition that I would personally add to this would be that of Echinacea to the twice daily garlic dose so as to try to stop the condition from getting worse. Consider the following Actions, Anti Catarrhal, Pectoral and if the patient is running a temperature and maybe a bit feverish consider the Actions of the Febrifuges and Diaphoretics but only if the symptoms match or so as to prevent the condition from getting worse.

Homoeopathic Treatment

Aconitum 6C - Early stages when mucous membrane of the nose is hot and dry, animal thirsty and feverish. Dose hourly for 4 doses.

Arsenicum Alb 1M - Discharge is acrid, swollen eyelids, thirst for small quantities, restless, worse after midnight. Dose every 2 hours for 4 doses.

Allium Cepa 6C - Discharge bland and watery, eyes red and watery and showing photophobia. Dose hourly for 4 doses.

Hepar Sulph 200C - Sneezing with ulceration of the nostrils, discharge thick and purulent, foul smelling, sensitive to pain, resents cold wind. Dose 3 times daily for 2 days.

Nat Mur 1M - Discharge whitish, albuminous looking, there may be violent sneezing, Dose every 2 hours for 4 doses.

Pulsatilla 30C - Loose cough, discharge of greenish fetid matter from nose, sneezing, often worse in morning, affectionate personality. Dose 3 times daily for 3 days.

Influenza

Equine influenza is caused by two strains of the Type A Influenza virus and are named after the cities where they were first found. The virus gains entry through the nose and attacks the linings of the trachea and bronchioles. The incubation period is about 3 to 4 days. This disease is highly contagious and can spread rapidly from horse to horse. In its pure state it consists of first a fever and secondly a specific affection of the mucous membranes of the upper respiratory tract and eyes. It most commonly affects young horses and appears usually in spring and autumn.

Signs and Symptoms - Febrile signs first appear and the temperature can go up to 41 degrees Celsius, the animal is dull and listless. There is a fast thready pulse, urine may be scanty and highly colored, the congestive swelling of the nose extends down the respiratory tract giving at first mucoid and later a purulent discharge. There can be copious and incessant discharge from the eyes and nose. The mouth can be sweaty and foul smelling often showing inflamed gums and inner cheeks, the coat is staring and breathing can be labored. The cough is harsh and dry and may develop early, the breathing is accelerated. The nervous system is also affected by a state of general languor and muscular weakness. The conjunctivae are discolored yellowish brown. For this condition mainly look for high fever, depression and cough along with a fast spread to other horses.

Herbal Treatment

Complete rest is essential for the body needs time to repair the damage especially to the mucous membranes. Treat the same as the common cold but increase the dosage of Garlic to 3 times a day. A wad of cotton wool should be dipped into warm water and a generous amount of Eucalyptus oil applied and with this the area of the lungs should be well massaged and then the body should be covered with a light weight blanket. The facial areas where there is congestion should also be massaged with the Eucalyptus oil in solution, 20 drops of oil to 1 tablespoon of hot water. Finally a half teaspoon full of Eucalyptus oil can be mixed with a tablespoon full of stiff honey or treacle and this paste then smeared over the tongue three times daily.

Following the 2 days fast (or longer if high fever continues) the diet should be laxative consisting mainly of bran mashes with molasses to which can be added chopped onion. Also a abundance of pulped carrots should be feed plus green food and sweet hay. Give a teaspoon full of Paprika daily preferably made into pills with flower and honey to check the burning properties till swallowed. In cases of great debility after influenza a nightly drench of ale (Guinness like beer - black) fortified with brown sugar or molasses. Our first consideration must be to build up the immune system and to attack the virus. We will use Echinacea for building up the immune system to this we will add Pau D Arco mainly for its Anti-Viral

Action which will add to that same action in Garlic. Our main problem here is that we have to watch out for and try to prevent secondary infections. The two most important Actions that we need for this condition are that of the Expectorants and Diaphoretics.

Try to double and triple your actions needed when making up herbal formulas, here Elder would be a good herb to use as the main Diaphoretic because all its other actions will help. Elder is virtually a specific for the flu.

Homoeopathic Treatment

Aconitum 6C - Early stages when febrile signs accompany anxious expression. Dose every hour for 4 hours.

Belladonna 200C - Acute cases, with full pulse, dilated pupils, skin hot and shiny, excitement and head shaking. Dose every hour for 4 doses.

Gelsemium 1M - Languor, muscular weakness, in coordination of movement. Dose every 2 hours for 4 doses.

Bryonia 6C - Harsh dry cough, pleuritic symptoms such as pain over chest and friction sounds are herd on auscultation. Relief on pressure, short grunting breathing. Dose 3 times daily for 3 days.

Ant Tart 30C - Saliva appears accompanied by moist cough and the presence of mucous rales on auscultation. Dose night and morning for 4 days.

Phosphorus 200C - Breathing short and rapid, pneumonia threatening. Dose 3 times daily for 2 days.

Arsenicum Alb 1M - Symptoms generally worse towards or after midnight, animal restless, drinks frequent small quantities, great weakness, skin dry and staring. Dose every 2 hours for 4 doses.

Bronchitis

Inflammation of the bronchial mucous membrane may arise independently of other illnesses or may be a sequel to influenza or catarrhal states. The condition can be more a broncho-pneumonia then a pure bronchitis. It may arise simply by exposure to cold dry winds or to damp and cold another aggravating factor can be dust and dusty living conditions.

Signs and Symptoms - Breathing is accelerated, pulse becomes full and quick accompanied by a frequent painful cough. Mucous secretion soon becomes purulent and may run from the nose as well as appear in the cough. Rattling respiratory sounds can be heard over the rib area.

Herbal Treatment

The treatment is treated fairly much the same as Colds and Influenza but we concentrate on the Actions of the Expectorants, Anti-inflammatories and Demulcents especially when there are signs of pain with the cough. Here are a list of some other Herbs that are very good for the treatment of bronchitis - Coltsfoot, Horehound, Licorice, Mullein, Pleurisy Root and White Horehound. If the cough is unproductive and causing pain think of Wild Cherry Bark which will act upon the nerve to stop the cough.

Also consider boosting the immune system because raw and damaged mucous tracts are very prone to secondary infections. I would also give a large dose of Vitamin C every day.

Another thing we can do is to make a steam bag by half filling a sack with bran or sawdust (pine sawdust is the best) then we make a hole in one side of the sack half way down so that hot water can be poured on to the bran or sawdust and to allow a little air to mix with the steam. One tablespoon of Eucalyptus oil can be poured on to the bran-sawdust. Thoroughly soak the contents of the bag with boiling water so a fierce steam is caused to rise. Apply the bag 3 times daily and be careful not to burn the horse.

Homoeopathic Treatment

Aconite 6C - Early stages, with hot dry skin, feverish symptoms and anxious expression. Dose hourly for 4 doses

Belladonna 1M - Pulse full and bounding, with dilated pupils, sweating and excitement. Dose every 2 hours for 4 doses.

Ant Tart 30C - Moist cough with threatened pulmonary edema, Rattling sounds may be herd in the chest, respirations increased. Dose 3 times daily for 3 days.

Bryonia 6C - Cough hard and dry, pleura becomes effected, relief from pressure over the ribs. Dose 3 times daily for 3 days.

Dulcamara 6C - Condition has origins from damp surroundings and coughing worse after exertion.

Dose 3 times daily for 3 days.

Kali Bich 200C - Phlegm in bronchial tubes difficult to expel, nasal discharge. Dose 3 times daily for 3 days.

Drosera 6C - Coughing becomes spasmodic in character, paroxysms follow one another rapidly. Dose 3 times daily for 4 days.

Spongia 6C - Bouts of coughing eased by eating or drinking, worse by exposure to cold air. Dose 3 times daily for 4 days.

Pneumonia

Inflammation of the lung tissue may appear as a result of overwork or chill and also as a sequel to diseases such as Influenza and Bronchitis. This is a serious condition that can lead to death.

Signs and Symptoms - Frequent pulse rate with discolored conjunctivae, followed by labored breathing and anxious or distressed look. As the condition progresses heaving on the flanks take place and the neck becomes extended as the animal seeks to take in more air. Legs and ears become cold and the mucous membranes of the nose and mouth assume a dusky dark bluish tinge. Cough may be blood stained or the mucous brought up rust colored.

Herbal Treatment

This is similar to the treatment of Influenza and Bronchitis so read those sections; our main herbs there are Echinacea and Garlic which are our main infection fighters. Looking at the fever side some good herbs to use from our Diaphoretics here are Yarrow, Elder and Hyssop. A effective formula could be Echinacea, Garlic, Ginger, Elder and Yarrow at about 20% of the formula each but make your formula to match the symptoms. The Eucalyptus nose bag may offer relief for this condition as well. Also consider the Anti-Catarrhal herbs and the Expectorants but realize with this condition you could be in trouble. Ensure lots of rest, warmth and lots of liquid which I would load with Vitamin C and a non-processed honey.

Homoeopathic Treatment

Aconite 6C - Should always be given first. Dose every half hour for 6 doses.

Bryonia 6C - Cough hard and dry, worse on movement and pressure over chest relieves, breathing is difficult and a grunting sound can sometimes be herd with each breath. Dose 3 times daily for 2 days.

Phosphorus 200C - A main remedy once hepatisation has set in, pressure resented particularly on the left side, sputum is rust colored, trembling of the body.

Iodum 30C - Hepatisation spreads rapidly, full pulse, absence of pain over chest, temperature remains high, sputum blood streaked. Dose every hour for 4 doses.

Sulphur 30C - Expectoration becomes greenish and purulent, pulse rate decreases towards evening and rises again later in the evening. Dose 3 times daily for 3 days.

Pleurisy

Injuries to the chest may lead to pleurisy and it may also arise from exposure to cold and damp but most of the time it comes from a lung infection or Pneumonia.

Signs and Symptoms - A quick thready pulse precedes a bout of shivering, signs of pain over the chest are indicated by abdominal breathing. There are general febrile symptoms such as discoloration of the conjunctiva and quickened pulse, the expression is anxious, inspiration is difficult but expiration is accomplished without much trouble. Cough is short dry and hacking with pain, pressure over ribs causes resentment, sometimes the skin over the pleura area becomes thickened into folds. Occasionally edema of the pleural cavities occurs leading to increased respiratory distress.

Herbal Treatment

Pleurisy is a infection so we shall attack the infection directly with Echinacea and Garlic, fever can also be a large part of pleurisy so we will attack this symptom with the herbs that are called Diaphoretics which are herbs used for fevers, some of them are Yarrow, Peppermint and Elder. As there is a lot of pain with this condition we shall add some Demulcent (soothing Herbs) herbs which will hopefully sooth the effected membranes and reduce the pain, a good one here to use is Mullein and I would also be inclined to add Coltsfoot for its all-round effect. For the Anti-Inflammatory herbs it would be a toss-up between

Comfrey and Golden Rod as these are both good all round herbs and their actions cover most of the symptoms of this disease. Also have a good look at the herb called Pleurisy Root. So a possible good formula we could make would be Echinacea, Garlic, Mullein, Yarrow and Comfrey at about 20% each so it is easy to make up. Try to make your formulas no more than five herbs at a time and try to base them on the actions you need. Always consider the pain side of this condition as it can cause extreme pain.

Homoeopathic Treatment

Aconite 6C - The early febrile stage. Dose hourly for 4 doses.

Bryonia 30C - Better at rest, pressure over pleural area relieves, cough usually hard and dry. Dose every 2 hours for 4 doses.

Apis 30C - Oedema occurs in pleural cavities, urine scanty and high colored. Dose 3 times daily for 3 days

Cantharis 200C - Pleural effusion, mucous expectorated with cough is usually blood stained, severe straining when trying to pass urine.

Kali Carb 200C - Symptoms of pain worse on right side, cough worse in early morning and there is usually a dry throat. Dose 3 times daily for 3 days.

Sulphur 6C - Use in the convalescent stage of pleurisy. Dose once daily for 6 days.

Strangles

Strangles is caused by the bacteria Streptococcus equi with a incubation period of 3 to 14 days and is the most important infectious disease problem for Australian horses. The disease is usually acute and is characterized by upper respiratory tract inflammation together with abscess formation in the glands below the jaw. Young animals are principally affected and the disease is highly contagious from horse to horse. Diseased horses should be isolated from the others. Paddocks and barn facilities used by infected horses should be regarded as contaminated for up to 2 months after resolution of an outbreak.

Signs and Symptoms - The first sign of infection is fever (103-106°F [39.4-41.1°C] and nasal discharge at first mucoid but soon becoming purulent and seen as a thick yellow discharge from the nose. Appetite is lost and the horse looks depressed. Throat involvement is usual in the form of an acute lymphadenitis. A persistent moist cough is present in most cases. The temperature is high in the initial stages and usually falls in 2 or 3 days but may reoccur once the abscesses develop in the throat glands. These become hot, swollen and tender to touch. Accompanying this abscess formation is a increase in purulent nasal discharge. The abscesses may rupture discharging a thick creamy pus. Extension to neighboring lymph glands is the rule in severe cases while accumulation of pus in the guttural pouches can result in neglected cases. Complications can be pneumonia and arthritis but few die of this disease.

Herbal Treatment

Garlic and Echinacea are our main herbal infection

fighters and to these I would be inclined to add Sage and Thyme as these herbs work well in the throat area. The following is copied from a old horse herbal. Fasting and general internal cleansing with heavy dosage of Garlic and laxative brews. Externally a nose bag should be used (see bronchitis) using steaming bran with a little Eucalyptus oil added. The purpose of the bag is to keep the nostrils well open by steaming. Should the tumor or tumors break internally this will be a great service. The breaking of tumors externally should not be attempted by poulticing because poultices can when cold act as a repellent to the opening of the tumors and thus retard the cure. The hair on all sides of the throat and jaw area should be clipped closely and the throat and tumors between the jaws massaged 3 times daily with a liniment made from finely cut Garlic COLD BREWED in turpentine - cold brew for 4 to 6 hours in a closed container shaking well every now and again. Approximately 3 good sized whole roots (not merely the cloves) of Garlic to one cupful of turpentine. The nostrils should be kept well sponged out with a water brew of Garlic or Elder or both. I would add Eucalyptus oil to the liniment.

Actions to consider are that of the Anti-Catarrhal and Diaphoretic Herbs. Some herbs used for Abscesses are Burdock, Cleavers, Coltsfoot, Echinacea, Fenugreek, Garlic and Myrrh. Be sure to match your Actions to the symptoms you are seeing and alter the formula as the symptoms change.

Homoeopathic Treatment

Aconite 6C - Always the first choice remedy in the early febrile stages. If given early enough this remedy alone may abort the disease. Dose hourly for 4 doses.

Belladonna 1M - Full bounding pulse, dilated pupils, nervous excitability. Dose every 2 hours for 4 doses.

Phytolacca 30C - Neighboring lymph glands or salivary glands in the throat becomes firm, tender and swollen. Dose 3 times daily for 4 days.

Pulsatilla 6C - Yellow mucous discharge from the nose, pharyngeal area tender, if the horse is a gentle mare give in a higher potency. Dose night and morning for 3 days.

Mercurius Sol 200C - Salivation and possibly slimy diarrhea, nasal discharge greenish and oily possibly blood stained. Dose night and morning for 3 days.

Hepar Sulph 200C - Low potencies will help the abscesses to ripen while in the higher potencies it will abort the rupture of the abscess. Dose low potency eg 6X three times daily for one day, higher potency night and morning for 2 days.

Herbal Overview Of The Respiratory System

Always start off with Echinacea and Garlic as you never know how violent the condition will become as this can save problems latter, also consider fasting the animal. Below are the Actions to think of when dealing with the Respiratory System. As usual isolate the animal and observe. Consider also if the condition is effecting another system ?. Is there diarrhea, is there any unusual behavior, is there fever, what is the temperature, is the animal anxious etc. Some of the best herbs for this system are Coltsfoot, Comfrey, Elder, Eyebright, Fenugreek, Golden Rod, Hyssop, Horehound, Horse Radish, Liquorice, Mullein, Myrrh, Plantain, Sage and Thyme.

Herbal Actions Of The Respiratory System

Anti-biotic - Echinacea, Garlic, Myrrh, Pau D Arco

Anti-catarrhal - Helps the body to remove excess catarrhal build ups.

Herbs - Coltsfoot, Cranesbill, Echinacea, Elder, Eyebright, Garlic, Golden Rod, Hyssop, Marshmallow, Mullein, Myrrh, Peppermint, Sage, Thyme, Yarrow.

Anti-inflammatory - Helps the body to combat inflammations. Herbs mentioned under demulcents will often act in this way especially when they coat sore throats and pipe lines.

Herbs - Comfrey, Cranesbill, Eyebright, Feverfew, Ginger, Golden Rod, Ladys Mantle, Liquorice.

Anti-microbial - Helps the body destroy or resist pathogenic micro-organisms.

Herbs - Aniseed, Echinacea, Garlic, Myrrh, Peppermint, Plantain, Rosemary, Sage, Thyme.

Antispasmodic - Prevents or eases spasms and

cramps.

Herbs - Aniseed, Coltsfoot, Fennel, Horehound, Hyssop, Mullein, Rosemary, Sage, Skullcap, Thyme

Anti-viral - Astragalus, Echinacea, Garlic, Myrrh?, Shitake, St Johns Wort, Pau D'Arco.

Anthelmintic - Destroys or expels worms from the digestive system.

Herbs - Garlic, Tansy, Wormwood, Thyme, Rue.

Astringent - Contracts tissue which in turn reduces discharges, these herbs contain tannins.

Herbs - Comfrey, Eyebright, Golden Rod, Marshmallow, Mullein, Myrrh, Plantain, Sage, Rosemary, Shepherds Purse, Thyme.

Demulcent - Soothes and protects irritated or inflamed internal tissues.

Herbs - Coltsfoot, Comfrey, Fenugreek, Liquorice, Marshmallow, Mullein, Oats, Plantain.

Diaphoretic - Aids the skin in the elimination of toxins and produces sweat thus reducing the temperature of fevers.

Herbs - Elder, Elecampane, Fennel, Garlic, Ginger, Golden Rod, Hyssop, Peppermint, Thyme, Yarrow.

Expectorant - Supports the body in the removal of excess mucous from the respiratory system and helps in the control of coughs.

Herbs - Aniseed, Coltsfoot, Comfrey, Elder, Elecampane, Fennel, Fenugreek, Garlic, Hyssop, Horehound, Liquorice, Marshmallow, Mullein, Myrrh, Plantain, Thyme.

Febrifuge - Helps the body to bring down fevers.

Herbs - Elder Flowers, Hyssop, Marigold, Penny Royal, Peppermint, Plantain, Raspberry, Sage, Thyme, Vervain.

Immune Booster - Astragalus, Echinacea, Pau D Arco

Pectoral - Has a general strengthening and healing effect on the respiratory system.

Herbs - Aniseed, Coltsfoot, Comfrey, Elder, Garlic, Hyssop, Liquorice, Mullein, Horehound.

The Reproductive System

Cystic Ovaries

Associated with the over development of the Graffian Follicle. In animals developing cystic ovary disease, ovulation fails to occur and the dominant follicle continues to enlarge. Moreover, other follicles may grow and form multiple cysts. The size and form of an affected ovary depends on how extensive the condition is. This condition can lead to one extreme or the other eg never coming to heat or even nymphomania. Between these conditions there could be irregular heat periods. Mares with this condition can show an uncertain temperament. The problem basically is a massive hormone imbalance which won't go away till the cysts stop developing. The bigger the cyst the more hormones it will be making. There may be a hereditary factor to this disease.

Signs and Symptoms - If the mare does not cycle there may be one or two cysts present. Symptoms can vary considerably. The condition is mainly diagnosed by rectal palpation where you can feel the cysts on the ovaries.

Herbal Treatment

This is difficult to treat so we will start with the basics. Think of starting off with Dong Quai , this is a specific for easing the pain of ovarian cysts but I want to use its blood cleansing properties (alterative) with those of Burdock which is also alterative but is also anti-tumor. What I am trying to do is focus on is cleansing out the womb and blood. We will have to run these herbs for at least 3 months as this is the time it takes for the blood to replace it self-e.g. the blood cycle. Another herb to think of adding to this is Black Cohosh as it is also a Alterative and is also used for pain. Think of using Chaste Tree in about 6 weeks after the first 2 two herbs have had a chance to clean up the area and hopefully reduce the size of the cysts as this will start having an action on the pituitary gland to start sorting out the hormone imbalances. If there is a lot of pain think of Wild Yam.

Homoeopathic Treatment

Apis 6C - One of the main remedies for dropiscal conditions. Used for swelling and puffing up of various parts, edema. Dose 3 time daily for 4 days.

Aurum Mur Nat 6C - When a chronic metritis is suspected and the whitish discharge shows. This remedy has a strong action on growths of the womb and surrounding areas. Ovaries may be indurated. Dose 3 times daily for 4 days.

Colocynth 6C - Nymphomania, multiple small cysts, great abdominal pain especially in the ovary area. Pains are relieved by pressure. Dose night and morning for 1 week.

Platina Met 30C - Nymphomania

Ovaritis

Inflammation of the ovaries can lead on to other problems especially if the condition spreads or becomes chronic. One problem that may result from this condition is adhesions.

Signs and Symptoms - There may be pain in the pelvic area with the mare kicking at one or the other flanks. The temperament may change with a docile mare becoming difficult.

Herbal Treatment

Here we need to find out what caused the ovaries to get inflamed in the first place. As mentioned in the above condition Dong Quai, Black Cohosh and Wild Yam are good for this condition especially for the pain. To these we need to add our immune booster and antibacterial herbs starting with Echinacea and Garlic. Also look at the anti-inflammatory herbs.

Homoeopathic Treatment

Aconite 6C - Give as soon as signs show especially when there is a raise in temperature, pulse and breathing. Dose hourly for 4 doses.

Apis 6C - One of the main remedies for dropiscal conditions. Used for swelling and puffing up of various parts, edema. Dose 3 time daily for 4 days.

Bryonia 6C - The right ovary is more effected with this remedy and the animal will prefer to lie on that side and may be still and quiet. Dose 3 times daily for 2 days.

Cimicifuga 30C - Left ovary affected, pains extend across lumber region and downwards towards udder, muscular and crampy like pains, nervousness. Dose night and morning for 4 days.

Lilium Tigrinum 200C - Accompanying signs of uterine inflammation such as discharges etc, discharges only when moving about, has a powerful influence over the pelvic organs, pain in ovaries and down thighs. Dose 3 times daily for 3 days.

Palladium 30C - Right ovary affected with leucorrhoea and flatulence, averse to exercise, pain seems to be relieved after stool and by rubbing. Dose night and morning for one week.

Contagious Equine Metritis (CEM)

This is an acute, highly contagious venereal disease of horses, characterized by a profuse, mucopurulent vaginal discharge and early return to estrus in most affected mares. Infected stallions and chronically infected mares show no clinical signs. The disease occurs primarily in Europe.

CEM is caused by the gram-negative, contagious equine metritis organism (CEMO). Important strain differences exist; some strains are resistant to streptomycin while others are streptomycin-sensitive. CEM is transmitted primarily at mating, but infected instruments and equipment also play a role. Undetected infected mares and stallions are the source of new outbreaks. Infected stallions show no signs and harbor the organism in the prepuce and the surface of the penis, especially in the urethral fossa. The transmission rate is exceptionally high; virtually every mare mated by an infected stallion becomes infected. . Chronically infected mares show no signs. Most mares do not conceive at the time of infected mating. If they do, they may infect the foal at or shortly after birth. Foals so infected may become carriers of CEMO when they reach sexual maturity.

Signs And Symptoms

Metritis in the early stages usually shows signs of fever and toxicity. Pulse and breathing are increased and sweating is common. In mares, a copious, mucopurulent vaginal discharge is seen 10-14 days after infected mating. Mares may return to estrus after a shortened estrous cycle. Although the discharge subsides after a few days, mares may remain infected for several months. This condition can lead to abortions and sterility in its chronic stage.

Homoeopathic Treatment

Strep Nosode 30C - Always start treatment with this remedy. Dose 3 times daily for 3 days.

Aconitum 6C - Should be given at the onset of the acute infection. Dose hourly for 4 doses.

Echinacea 6X - Helps to fight the Strep in the blood stream. Dose every 2 hours for 4 doses.

Pyrogen 1M - Metritis resulting from abortion or retention of some of the afterbirth. This nosode is indicated when a weak thready pulse alternates with a high temperature or vice versa. The most useful remedy in septic conditions. Give every 2 hours for 4 doses.

Sabina 6C - Bleeding of bright red blood from uterus. Retained pieces of afterbirth. Dose every hour for 5 doses.

Belladonna 1M - The mare is excitable, sweating and hot skin. Indicated when the animal is hot to touch with a full bounding pulse and dilated pupils. Signs of cerebral excitement may be present with extreme cases convulsions. Give every hour for 5 hours.

Sepia 200C - Chronoc Metritis, uterine discharges. Dose weekly for 4 doses.

Before Pregnancy

The best ages for breeding in mares are from 3 to 14 years. Ensure the mare is fit and in good health. To improve chances of conceiving look at the herbal treatment under Infertility. Start the treatment with Chaste Tree and Raspberry at least 2 to 3 months before you intend to send the mare to stud.

Infertility

Some problems leading to infertility are Cystic Ovaries, Inflammation of the ovaries, Leucorrhoea, Endometritis (inflammation of the lining of the womb), Metritis (inflammation of the womb) and vaginitis. A lot of the problems just mentioned can be the result of infections. Problems of this nature need to be corrected before pregnancy can be expected. Other considerations can be structural defects in the vulva, hormone imbalance, nutritional factors, psychological problems and there can be lots of other things as well so this is the time to get a vet and see what is going on. Even in the racing industry 20 to 25% won't fall pregnant each season.

Herbal Treatment

Here we will leave the infections alone as some of

them are covered latter and just concentrate on the main hormone balancing herbs. The main balancing herb to think of here is Chaste Tree as this herb has a action on the pituitary gland. The pituitary gland is the master gland of the hormone system as this gland tells most of the other glands what to do and when, so this herb deals with the boss.

Chaste Tree has a stimulating and normalizing effect on the pituitary glands functions especially its progesterone function. The main use of this herb is for normalizing the activity of female hormones. Always think of the hormone progesterone as pro - pregnancy as one of the jobs of this hormone is to prepare the womb for the fertilized egg so the more of this hormone there is the thicker the lining of the womb will be greatly enhancing the survival of the egg. A good herb to use with Chaste Tree is Raspberry as it strengthens and tones the tissues of the womb and is a good tonic, together these two herbs cover a lot of problems.

Pregnancy

The mare should be kept in good physical condition and be receiving a good diet suitable for her condition along with gentle exercise. The term of pregnancy should be 340 days but could be anywhere from 15 days before to a month late. Signs of birthing becoming due are the udder beginning to fill which is usually 3 to 6 weeks before birth and the udder will get to its maximum size 6 to 48 hours before birth.

Another sign is that the muscles around the vulva become relaxed and soft as the body prepares for birth. All herbal supplements should be stopped once pregnancy has been achieved as a lot of herbs stimulate the uterus and may cause abortion especially in the early stages. Remember to treat the foals umbilical stump, tie up the afterbirth so the mare doesn't step on it and afterward when the afterbirth is finally expelled make sure it is all there. I will keep this section short as there is lots of information out there.

Herbal Treatment

Raspberry leaf is the most important herbal aid to a easy birth as it tones the uterine muscles, is very high in vitamins and minerals and increases and enriches the milk production. Another important reason for using Raspberry is because of its high astringency which gives us protection against excessive bleeding. Raspberry should be given to all breeders especially the ones that have had difficult births before and those that have had retained after birth before. Give Raspberry before pregnancy and in the last couple of months before birth. Herbs to think of to increase the milk production are Fenugreek, and Fennel.

Homoeopathic Treatment

Viburnum Opulis - A remedy for use in the early stages of pregnancy up to one month to 6 weeks. Helps to eliminate the tendency to early miscarriage. Give 30C three times per week for 4 weeks.

Caulophyllum - This remedy is used for the latter

stages. Helps to ensure a trouble free birth and tones up the uterus for easy expulsion of the afterbirth. Give 30C three times per week for the last 4 weeks. If the last stage of labor is delayed or weak this remedy should be given again to help speed up normal contractions.

Arnica 30C - This can be used at the time of birthing and given for a few days after as it will help with the bruising and swelling and is good for shock. Give 3 times a day.

BellisPerennis 30C - If the birthing was prolonged or severe give this remedy along with Arnica.

Post Birth Problems
Retained Placenta

I used to have an area for birthing and one of the most important reasons for this is that you would always know if the afterbirth had been expelled. The first thing you should do after birth is to get the foal to suckle as this is the main trigger to release the after birth. The afterbirth form a horse is very large especially when taking the sack into consideration but it is very important you put it together again like a jigsaw puzzle so you can be sure that all of it has been expelled from the womb if it hasn't an infection will probably result.

Herbal Treatment

Juliette de Bairacli Levy recommends to keep fasting the mare and then give a quart strong brew of 3 parts Raspberry leaf to 1 part Feverfew strengthened with molasses. All of these substances are stimulating and tonic to the womb. Another herb to think of is Pennyroyal which is virtually the specific for this condition.

Homoeopathic Treatment

Homoeopathic remedies to consider are Sepia 30C, Pulsatilla 6c, Satilla 6C and Pyrogen 1M.

Sabina - Useful when the condition is associated with the retention of the afterbirth or miscarriage especially in those cases showing blood stained discharges. Give 6C every hour for 6 doses.

Hemorrhage

Herbal Treatment

Give internally via the mouth a strong infusion of about 600mls of Raspberry. Astringents are the main herbs that you use to stop bleeding. Two of the strongest ones are Shepherds Purse and Cranesbill. Make a 1 to 10 lotion of either of these herbs and if bleeding cannot be controlled use a small syringe without the needle to gently inject into the womb, hopefully this will spasm the ends of the bleeding vessels and stop the flow of blood. For less severe bleeding we can use a lotion of our main first aid remedy Calendula. It would also be wise to clean the whole area with Calendula for its antibacterial and wound healing actions.

Homoeopathic Treatment

This does not occur to often but when it does try to match one of the remedies below.

Ipecacuanah 6C - Blood accumulates in the uterus and is then expelled in a bright red flood. Give every hour for 5 doses.

Crotalus 1M - If the blood comes away as a steady drip. Give every hour for 4 doses.

Hammamelis 30C - Dark blood indicating a venous origin will need this remedy. Give 1 dose every 2 hours up to 5 times.

Secale 30C - Very stringy blood indicates this remedy. Give 1 dose every 2 hours up to 5 times.

Metritis Acute

Metritis or inflammation of the womb can be acute or chronic. The acute condition is associated with the birth and is usually a bacterial invasion of the lining of the womb. Chief among the causes of this condition is the retained placenta or pieces of it together or with infection which gains entrance to the genital tract. Abortions can cause this condition as well.

Signs and Symptoms - This usually occurs 24 hours after birthing. There is a rise in temperature followed by a loss of appetite and the mare is uneasy and lethargic. Respirations are increased and there may be a expression of anxiety on the face, abdominal pains, coma. Inflammation of the uterus may travel down to the vulva and vagina making them inflamed and dark red. Discharge is not always present but if it is it may vary from a yellowish color through to blood stained.

Herbal Treatment

We will start off by telling you how this problem on the pregnancy side could of probably been avoided in the first place. If the mare was given the herb Raspberry in the last months of pregnancy the womb would of been toned and strengthened and the problem may of been avoided. When the foal is born it is usually when they start to suckle that triggers the expulsion of the placenta. Inflammations of the uterus arising from infection should be treated with the main immune boosting herbs mainly Echinacea, Garlic and another good one if you have got it is Myrrh. To these herbs consider adding Ladys Mantle (astringent) and Black Cohosh. Dong Qua could also be added to the Black Cohosh as these are both Alteratives and pain killers. A lotion of Calendula could be used to clean the outside area especially if it is red and sore also think of adding Hypericum to the lotion for pain relief.

Homoeopathic Treatment

Treatment should be started as bad signs start to appear after parturition especially after a dead foal and a difficult labor.

Aconitum 1M - Should be given at once so as to quickly allay shock, fear and anxiety and regulate the circulation. Give every hour for 4 hours.

Belladonna 1M - Indicated when the animal is hot to touch with a full bounding pulse and dilated pupils. Signs of cerebral excitement may be present with extreme cases convulsions. Give every hour for 5 hours.

Lillum Tig 30C - A good general remedy for uterine congestion leading to blood stained discharges and straining in the pelvic region.

Secale 30C- Hemorrhages are present when this remedy is considered, the blood is fluid and dark, the patient is cadaverous looking with cold extremities which are deficient in blood supply. Give twice daily for 10 days.

Sabina 6C- Useful when the condition is associated with the retention of the afterbirth or miscarriage especially in those cases showing blood stained discharges. Give every hour for 6 doses.

Pyrogen 1M - This nosode is indicated when a weak thready pulse alternates with a high temperature or vice versa. The most useful remedy in septic conditions. Give every 2 hours for 4 doses.

Mastitis

The cause can be a combination of factors such as exposure to cold winds and wet weather, injuries from blows and sharp objects, insufficient stripping of the udder in milking and bacterial infections caught from others. Acute mastitis occurs occasionally in lactating mares, most commonly in the drying-off period, in one or both glands. Streptococcus zooepidemicus is the most frequent form.

Signs and Symptoms - Check the mare frequently just after weaning. Marked painful swelling of the affected gland and surrounding tissues are signs of mastitis, fever and depression may be present. The mare may walk stiffly or stand with the hind legs apart due to the discomfort from the inflammation. Run a little milk off and if it appears lumpy and yellow in color it probably is mastitis.

Herbal Treatment

Photolacca (Poke Root) tincture in small doses is the main herb for mastitis though I believe the Homoeopathic potency is far better and faster acting then the tincture. Care must be taken with this herb only use in small doses. To the Homoeopathic Dose you could make a lotion for external application of Photolacca but make it a very mild lotion as this is a strong remedy so make it about 1 to 20 in strength. The main immune boosting and anti-bacterial herbs should also be used these are Echinacea and Garlic. In the past Wood Sage and Garlic used to be the specific for this condition.

Pat Coleby says to give 3 table spoons of dolomite and sodium ascorbate in her feed daily until the symptoms ease. In serious cases give a intramuscular injection of Troys injectable Vitamin C.

Homoeopathic Treatment.

Common frequent remedies used on a individual basis are as below.

Aconite 6X - This should be used as routine in all acute cases especially in those that develop suddenly, it will allay tension and restlessness, cause may be from exposure from cold dry winds. Dose every half hour for 6 doses.

Arnica 30C - Indicated when mastitis develops as a result of injury to the mammary tissue, blood may be present in the milk. Dose 3 times daily for 3 days.

Apis 6C - This is a useful remedy for freshly birthed mares showing edema of the udder and surrounding tissues. The mammary vein is usually engorged in this case. Dose every 3 hours for 4 doses.

Belladonna 1M - Indicated usually in the acute form post-partum. The udder shows acute swelling and redness, pain is obvious on touch, the animal will feel hot with full bounding pulse. Dose every hour for 4 doses.

Bryonia 30C - Indicated where the udder swelling is hard and indurated. In acute cases pain will be relieved by pressure on the udder and such cases are frequently presented with the animal lying down as this appears to give relief. Chronic forms showing fibrosis should benefit from this remedy. Dose 4 hourly for 4 doses while in the chronic form dose twice weekly for a month.

Phytolacca 30C - A useful remedy for both acute and chronic cases. Acute form may show curdled milk and clots while in the latter small clots may appear in mid lactation. This is probably the most useful remedy for the average chronic case. Dose 3 times daily for 3 days followed once daily for 4 days.

Urtica Urens 6X - For acute forms showing edema which may be in the form of plaques frequently extending to the perineal area. Dose every hour for 4 doses.

Hepar Sulph 6X - This low potency will help promote

suppuration and clearing of the udder contents in cases of C. Pyogenes or summer mastitis infection. Dose every 3 hours for 4 doses. Once the udder has been cleared of purulent material a dose or 2 of a higher potency should be given to complete the cure.

Ipecac 30C - This is a useful remedy for controlling intra-mammary bleeding which results in pink milk. Dose 3 times daily for 3 days.

Teats Sore Or Damaged

The delicate tissues of the teat sometimes become chapped and may develop deep fissures.

Signs and Symptoms - The Mare will not tolerate the foal feeding. Do a visual examination of the area and check out for swelling and mastitis.

Herbal Treatment

Juliette de Bairacli Levy recommends to treat alternately with warm almond oil as a salve and bathed with a brew of equal parts elder blossom and marshmallow. Raw cucumber juice has been effective. I would use Calendula and Hypericum Lotion (1 to 10) as this is a great healer of all wounds and also helps to relieve the pain. Calendula is well known for closing wounds fast and the Hypericum will help with the sharp pains of this area. Clean with lotion and then apply the same as a cream.

Herbal Overview Of The Reproductive System

The right way of using herbs is to know all the actions and what they do, so the idea is that you train yourself to think in actions not in herbs. In this way you start to get an all-round picture of your patient without being blinded by your favorite herbs. Below are some of the actions to consider for this system. In the Astringents the herbs underlined are the best to use to stop bleeding; some are used more internally such as Ladys Mantle while others are used more externally such as Witch Hazel. Use the Alteratives for Chronic diseases of this system and maybe add some of the Emmenagogues to them so as to guide them where you want them to do the cleaning. With chronic diseases the rule is at least one month's treatment to every year the patient has had the disease. Read up on the individual herbs and use the ones that work in the direction you want and make your decisions after that. Always try to get clear in your head the actions you want and what you want to achieve by using them.

Herbal Actions For The Reproductive System

Alterative - Herbs that gradually restore proper function to the body, they increase health and vitality. They were once known as the blood cleansers.

Herbs - Black Cohosh, Dong Quai, Damiana. Burdock is good for tumors.

Anti-biotic - Echinacea, Garlic, Myrrh, Pau D' Arco, Burdock

Anti-fungal - Calendula, Cats Claw, Pau D' Arco, Myrrh, Sweet Violets.

Anti-inflammatory - Helps the body to combat inflammations. Herbs mentioned under demulcents, emollients and vulnerary's will often act in this way especially when they are applied externally.

Herbs - Chamomile, Feverfew, Ginger, Golden Rod, Ladys Mantle, Liquorice, Marshmallow, Meadowsweet, Calendula, Pau D' Arco.

Anti-Tumor - Burdock, Cleavers, Reshi, Shitake, Sweet Violets.

Antispasmodic - Prevents or eases spasms and cramps.

Herbs - Aniseed, Black Cohosh, Chamomile, Fennel, Hyssop, Motherwort, Rosemary, Rue, Sage, Thyme, Valerian, Vervain.

Anti-viral - Astragalus, Cats claw, Echinacea, Garlic, Myrrh?, Shitake, Pau D'Arco.

Astringent - Contracts tissue which in turn reduces discharges, these herbs contain tannins.

Herbs - Cranesbill, Ladys Mantle, Calendula, Raspberry, Shepherds Purse, Witch Hazel.

Emmenagogue - Stimulates and normalizes the menstrual flow, tonics for the female reproductive system.

Herbs - Black Cohosh, Chamomile, Fenugreek, Gentian, Ginger, Ladys Mantle, Marigold,

Motherwort, Parsley Peppermint, Parsley, Raspberry, Sage, Rosemary, Rue, Shepherds Purse, Tansy, Thyme, Valerian, Vervain, Yarrow.

Galactagogue - Helps increase the flow of milk in females.

Herbs - Aniseed, Fennel, Fenugreek, Milk Thistle, Raspberry, Vervain.

Notes

The Nervous System

Encephalitis

This term implies inflammation of the brain or any inflammatory lesion occurring to the brain tissue. It leads to loss of nervous function. There can be many causes for this condition and often it is fatal.

Signs and Symptoms - Encephalitis is usually accompanied by fever, toxemia, anorexia, depression and tachycardia. Normal stimuli can produce exaggerated responses, the animal being easily startled. There may be convulsions accompanied by squinting of eyes and clamping of jaws. Paresis and ataxia may precede paralysis. Most deaths occur 2 to 3 days after clinical signs are seen.

Herbal Treatment

Herbal treatment could be too slow for a fast acting disease as this but consider Garlic ,Echinacea and Myrrh for bacterial and viral infections. Another herb to look at is St Johns Wort because it is a Nervine anti-viral. Essential oils can cross the blood brain barrier and could be a fast way of getting into the area so try maybe Garlic oil ,Lavender oil, Myrrh, Thyme or Eucalyptus diluted and rubbed in the area as these are all anti-microbials. I have not heard of essential oils being used for this condition but as a last desperate resort I would try it. Consider L lysine as this increases interferon and may slow down viral replication. Upon recovery of the acute phase consider giving Astragalus and Oats as a tonic and to help repair any damage. Homoeopathy is the better action to take as it is faster acting then herbal medicine.

Homoeopathic Treatment

Aconite 6C - If seen early enough this should be given in the febrile stage.

Belladonna 1M - This remedy is useful for deranged nerve conditions, there is a accompanying full bounding pulse, fever, dilated pupils and a smooth hot skin. Dose hourly for 4 doses.

Stramonium 30C - Indicated when signs of vertigo appear, such as a tendency to stagger and fall sideways, the eyes are usually wide open and staring. Dose 4 times daily for 2 days.

Hyoscyamus 200C - Indications for this remedy include frequent head shaking and a tendency to muscular twitching. There may be signs of abdominal discomfort. Dose 3 times daily for 3 days.

Phosphorus 200C - Useful in less acute cases showing a tendency to reoccur. The animal becomes unsteady after rising. Dose night and morning for one week.

Zincum Met 6C - Indicated where there is a tendency for the head to roll from side to side. Hyperaesthesia and hyper-excitability are present, easily startled, paddling of feet may occur. Dose 3 times daily for 3 days.

Meningitis

Inflammation of the meninges is usually secondary to viral or bacterial infection. There is no specific cause of meningitis which is far more common in foals then in the adult horse. Infection may enter through a penetrating wound, but more often the infection is spread through the blood and in foals it can be from a infected naval.

Signs and Symptoms - This condition is characterized by fever and muscle rigidity. Sensitivity of the skin is a common symptom, there is a retraction of the head and stiffness of the neck muscles, paresis of the hindquarters is common. There can be increased nervous activity and so increased response to pain, excitement or depression and a raised body temperature.

Herbal Treatment

This is the same as Encephalitis. Meningitis is a fast acting acute infection and herbal remedies may act to slow to control the condition but would be very helpful in assisting the recovery.

The best action here is to call the vet and hope that he has the right antibiotics to target the cause.

Homoeopathic Treatment

Aconite 6C - Should be given in the early febrile stage, the animal usually looks anxious and there is a rapid short pulse. Dose hourly for 4 hours.

Belladonna 1M - The indications for this remedy are a accompanying encephalitis with dilated pupils and a throbbing pulse, the skin is smooth and hot, sweating is common. Dose 2 hourly for 3 doses.

Zincum Met 6C - Indicated where there is a tendency for the head to roll from side to side. Hyperaesthesia and hyper-excitability are present, easily startled, paddling of feet may occur. Dose 3 times daily for 3 days.

Bryonia 6C - Indicated in cases showing vertigo, the animal resents movement and there is excessive dryness of the mucous membranes e.g. seen in the mouth where the lips show a parched appearance and there is great thirst. Dose 3 times daily for 3 days.

Veratum 30C - The legs and ears are icy cold, there is convulsive trembling of the whole body or there is a reeling, staggering motion, and the animal plunges violently and falls down head foremost.

Cuprum Met 30C - A useful remedy when convulsions are associated more with meningitis then with encephalitis. The head usually assumes a lowered posture and there may be attempts to press it against any suitable object.

Epilepsy

This is largely hereditary in horses. Because of the nature of the horses work this disease is always a source of danger to the owner as the sudden falling down of the animal, which is the chief symptom of the disease and the wild uncontrollable kicking that follows has often caused serious accidents.

Signs and Symptoms - These may start off as minor convulsions which last sometimes less than a minute and usually do not have a loss of consciousness with them. These attacks tend to become more serious but less frequent as the animal gets older. Attacks can come on suddenly without any symptoms or there may be symptoms of restlessness or uneasiness prior to the seizure, afterwards the animal may be lethargic and sleepy looking. It is difficult to recognize a epileptic animal but sometimes you can see the scaring on the body especially the legs.

Herbal Treatment

You need to try to prescribe on the whole picture of the horse and it may be worthwhile adding oats to the diet as this is a good nerve food. Herbs that have been used for epilepsy are Skullcap which is one of the main remedies. Drench twice daily with a strong brew of Skullcap herb two handfuls of the herb brewed in 3 pints of water and one table spoon of honey added. Give one pint twice daily. Other useful herbs can be Vervain, Mistletoe, Gotu Kola, Hyssop and Passion Flower. To build up the nervous system and strengthen it think of Oats, Chamomile and Valerian. Concentrate more on the Nervine Restoratives.

Homoeopathic Treatment

If there has been a history of short attacks which pass off quickly the following remedies will help delay the onset of further seizures and will also help during the attack limiting it considerably.

Belladonna 30C - This is one of the most frequently indicated remedies, for attacks associated with dilated pupils and throbbing pulse, the animal will usually feel abnormally hot.

Stramonium 30C - This remedy is somewhat similar to the last one but there are usually signs before the fit such as staggering with a tendency to fall toward the left side, eyes are again dilated and staring.

Hyoscyamus 30C - Indicated when attacks are preceded by shaking of the head and a unsteadiness of gait indicating vertigo, there may be spasmodic closing of the eyelids and the mouth is flecked with foam.

Cocculus 6C - The main use for this remedy lies more in the preventative sphere and is useful to ward off subsequent attacks. It should be given at regular intervals over a period of a few months.

Ignatia 6C - Consciousness is usually lost when this remedy is indicated. The head may be shaken to and fro and this precedes hysterical turns.

Cuprum Met 30C - A useful remedy when convulsions are associated more with meningitis then with encephalitis. The head usually assumes a lowered posture and there may be attempts to press it against any suitable object.

Paralysis of the Facial Nerve

This is a fairly common occurrence in a horse and may be unilateral or bilateral. There are various causes including trauma and exposure to the cold. A toxic form may arise as a squeal to some infectious disease such as strangles or influenza.

Signs and Symptoms - When the condition is unilateral the lips are drawn to the side, bilateral involvement can effect eating and drinking as the lower lip hangs down. Occasionally the animal has difficulty in closing the eyelids.

Herbal Treatment

If disease brought on the condition consider Garlic ,Echinacea, Myrrh and St Johns Wort for bacterial and viral infections. If the cause was injury use St Johns Wort internally and externally as a lotion along with Calendula externally until wound is healed. The action to concentrate on here is the Nervine Restoratives especially oats. Latter consider the Nervine Stimulants especially if you have had no result, Guarana is the one to consider here as it has helped in paralysis before.

Homoeopathic Treatment

Gelsemium 200C - This is one of the main remedies in treating motor paralysis of various groups of muscles and nerves, it is especially useful if the paralysis is a squeal to infectious disease particularly influenza. Dose once daily for one week.

Causticum 30C - This remedy is particularly useful if the condition has arisen as a result of exposure to cold. Dose night and morning for 5 days.

Grass Sickness

This is a disease in which degeneration of the autonomic nervous system leads to paralysis of the whole digestive tract from the throat to the rectum. This condition is more commonly seen in animals 3 to 7 years though it can happen at any age. The condition happens to animals at grass especially ones that have just returned from winter stabling. This condition is mainly seen in Northern Europe but recently there has been a few cases in the USA. In acute cases the animal dies in one to 4 days. while in chronic cases they can last weeks to months. This is a non-infectious disease. As some fields are more associated with this condition then others it would be interesting if a soil analysis was taken and compared to other fields.

Signs and Symptoms - Symptoms are variable but will include the following. High pulse, sweating, muscular tremors accompanied by a rapid loss of condition. Difficulty in swallowing, food and water may fall from mouth and nose. Thirsty but cannot swallow and will hang around the trough and look as though playing with the water. Horse then becomes dehydrated and little urine is passed. Stomach becomes distended and bowel motions may cease or change and their may be severe and painful colic following.

Herbal Treatment

Juliette de Bairacli Levy treats this condition by giving a strong drench made of 2 handfuls of Sage leafs in one liter of water with aniseed and honey. Give alternate drenches of a strong brew of Poppy flower or heads, Hops or Lime blossom. Give 20 charcoal Tablest to absorb the inner fermentation. Externally apply to the bowels area and the whole belly area hot cloths rung out in a brew of Sage, Thyme or

Rosemary.

I would start treatment with a purge, go to the digestive system then to constipation and give the Senna purge , another purge to consider is castor oil as this empties the whole bowel but is a harsh purge. If we can get the contents of the digestive system out as fast as we can maybe we can minimize the cause of the problem and reduce the effect on the rest of the body. Another thing to consider is a coffee enema. After this I would consider the Charcoal tablets mentioned above. Concentrate on the Stimulant herbs start with Guarana which is a slow release form of caffeine and a specific for paralysis which is why I mentioned it for a enema, give this with Oats in tincture form with Oats being a Nervine restorative and Stimulant. Next we will move on to Alterative Nervines which are the blood cleansers focused to the nervous system Gotu Kola, St Johns Wort and Black cohosh. Now let's consider the liver which has to detox all the toxins which may be part of the cause but will now have to clean up what our Nervine Alteratives are stirring up. The herb we shall use here is Vervain which has a affinity for the liver, nerves and digestive system. Next consider some digestive herbs with nervine actions with the best being Peppermint then maybe Chamomile and   Gentian is also worth considering as it is a digestive stimulant and is used for depression and melancholy. Look at the main herbs I have chosen and find their actions and you will see that I am using them for 3 to 4 or more of their actions, try to do the same. As there is no cure for this disease we can only learn and try and then pass on our knowledge.

Homoeopathic Treatment

Gelsemium 1M - In this high potency we may be able to get the horse to swallow. This is a good remedy for creeping paralysis and should be the one first considered.

Plumbum Met 30C - Generalized paralysis, especially of the gut, progressive muscular atrophy along with rapid emaciation and painful colic.

Conium - When hind leg paralysis occurs as in the sitting dog posture. This is more of a assending paralysis rather than a decending one so take this into consideration. If this picture fits use a high potency if not use at 30C.

Zincum Met 30C - Muscle tremors and patchy sweating, trembling, twitching, fidgety feet, abdomen distended.

Cocculus 30C - Associated with lower limb paralysis and distended abdomen with pain.

Nux Vom - For the irritable type of horse, bowels not moving and digestive problem, weakness and numbness of lower limbs. If symptoms match give in high potency.

Lathyrus - This remedy may help to restore nerve function if not already lost, paralytic affections of the lower extremities, tottering gait.

Thallium 30C - Paralysis of the lower limbs, pains in stomach and bowels, trembling, very tired.

Tetanus (Lock Jaw)

This disease is caused by the bacterium Clostridium tetani gaining entrance to the body through a puncture or other deep wounds that are not exposed to the air. If this bacteria finds dead tissues and no oxygen it will multiply rapidly making a potent toxin which then circulates through the blood supply damaging the central nervous system. High risk injuries are puncture wounds of the hoofs, stake wounds and deep thorn penetrations.

Signs and Symptoms - Clinical signs are most often observed 2 weeks after a injury occurs. The animal walks in a unsteady manner, there is muscle stiffness and muscular spasms, very erect and rigid ears, inability to open mouth (lock jaw). As the disease progresses the stiffness gets more severe and the breathing becomes rapid and shallow. Severe cases involve the central nervous system with convulsions and death from respiratory failure.

Herbal Treatment

The main herb to think of here is Hypericum also known as St Johns Wort. This herb is used as a nervine anti-viral and bacterial. Traditionally it has been used to help prevent tetanus especially in horses that have trodden on a nail that has gone through the fetlock. The treatment for horses was to pour straight tincture into the wound in the hope it would kill the bacteria. Treat all wounds with Hypericum and Calendula tinctures mixed half and half diluted with water. See the Animal First Aid Book. For this condition Pat Coleby says if you suspect tetanus tap the horse smartly under the chin and the eyes will roll back and eventually the jaw will lock. In this case she says to immediately give a 50ml inramuscular injection of Vitamin C and repeat every 2 hours until the horse improves.

Homoeopathic Treatment

The following remedies may give some relief and in mild cases and may lead to cure especially if started early.

Acconitum 10M - For the fear and anxiety, always give at the first signs of a problem. Give every hour for 4 doses.

Curare 30C - Helps where muscle stiffness is prominent. Give three times daily for 7days.

Strychninum 200C - The arching of the back together with extension of limbs and head matches the symptoms of this remedy. Give twice daily for 3 days.

Hypericum 1M - This remedy may help in limiting the spread of the toxin. Give three times daily for 7 days.

Ledum 6C - This is the main remedy for puncture wounds especially if they feel cold. Give frequently in the potency.

Tetanus Nosode - Combine the nosode with the selected remedy. Use for 7 days in the 30th potency.

Herbal Overview Of The Nervous System

One of the most important herbs in this system is Hypericum also known as St Johns Wort. This herb is anti-viral, antibacterial, anti-inflammatory, a sedative and one of our main first aid remedies for wounds which helps relieve pain and can kill the tetanus bacteria and this is only mentioning a part of its uses, always consider this when there are problems with this system especially if you don't know what the problem is. Another good herb for rebuilding this system is Oats which is a Nervine tonic also think of Valerian which is our main Tranquillizer but also a good tonic for this system. A lot of the herbs mentioned below are used in a lot of other body systems as well so when you want the action of a Nervine to use in another system try to match the herb to one used in that system as well.

Herbal Actions Of The Nervous System

Antispasmodic - Prevents or eases spasms and cramps.

Herbs - Aniseed, Angelica, Black Cohosh, Chamomile, Fennel, Horehound, Hyssop, Lime Blossom, Mistletoe, Motherwort, Rosemary, Rue, Sage, Skullcap, St johns Wort, Thyme, Valerian, Vervain.

Anodynes - These are pain killing herbs.

Herbs - Black Cohosh, Jamician Dogwood, St Johns Wort, Valerian, Wild Yam, Wood Betony

Nervine - Has a beneficial effect on the nervous system, acts like a tonic to this system.

Herbs - Black Cohosh, Chamomile, Hops, Lime Blossoms, Mistletoe, Motherwort, Oats, Peppermint, Rosemary, Skullcap, St Johns Wort, Tansy, Thyme, Valerian, Vervain, Wormwood.

Nervous Restoratives - Oats, Gotu Kola, Damiana, Bacopa, Vervain, Rosemary, Skullcap

Nervine Stimulants - Guarana, Coffee, Peppermint, Oats, Gotu Kola, Gingseng, St Johns Wort.

Sedative - Calms the nervous system and reduces stress and nervousness throughout the body.

Herbs - Black Cohosh, Chamomile, Hops, Hyssop, Motherwort, Skullcap, St Johns Wort, Valerian , Vervain.

The Urinary System

Nephritis (Kidney Inflammation)

With horses weakness of the kidneys is usually a heredity condition and those with the weakness are prone to problems in this area. Some causes of Nephritis can be by long exposure to cold and damp, or the carrying of over heavy weights on long distances, also over use of grain foods with their high content of calcium salts and some commercial feeds are not readily assimilated which places a heavy strain upon the kidneys and often prove directly irritating to the delicate internal kidney tissues. Streptococcal infection may be a contributory cause of this condition in a horse or any form of systemic blood infection especially if stones and gravel are present as they can cause a wound for the infection to enter.

Signs and Symptoms - The first noticeable sign may be a peculiar stiff and unnatural hind gait. The horse cannot tolerate pressure to the kidney area and there may be a constant attempt to void urine and the little that is passed is both thick and dark hued, there may be great thirst.

The main signs are diminished urine output compared to intake and threatened anuria (stoppage of urine) while in the latter stages uraemic (blood poisoning) signs appear including increased respirations, sleepiness, intermittent diarrhea and finally coma. Urine tests will be needed as sometimes there is blood in the urine and a high content of proteins which there shouldn't be. The acute stage is marked by swelling of the kidney together with tissue edema. Pain and tenderness over the kidney region is a fairly constant sign. Increased thirst may accompany the chronic form due to salt retention.

Herbal Treatment

Juliette de Bairacli Levy treats this condition by fasting and using the herbs Parsley, Chicory and Horsetail. Four handfuls of herb boiled and brewed in1 quart of water with 2 tablespoons of honey added when the brew has cooled to tepid. Other herbs to consider for kidney problems are Bearberry, Buchu and Corn silk. If you think the condition may of been caused by infection think of Echinacea and Garlic. Remember this is a life threatening problem and a vet should be called because there may have to be some very quick decisions made. Actions to consider for this condition are Anti Inflammatory, Demulcents and Urinary Antiseptics. The convalescent diet should include abundant steamed nettles and pulped carrots. Barley is the best cereal to be used for kidney cases, feed also couch grass.

Homoeopathic Treatment

Apis 6C - Renal oedema in the acute form, urine shows albuminous casts. Dose every 2 hours for 4 doses.

Arsenicum 6C- Scanty urine showing albumen content and drops of blood, the animal is restless and thirsty for small amounts, there is a harsh dry coat, symptoms are worse after midnight. Dose every

2 hours for 4 doses.

Belladonna 1M - Acute cases showing excitement and dilated pupils, full bounding pulse and hot smooth skin, straining to pass urine which is scanty and loaded with phosphates, blood in urine is common. Dose every 2 hours for 4 doses.

Mercurius Sol 30C - Urine scanty with greenish mucous sediment which may contain pus and blood. Urine is dark colored. Dose 3 times daily for 4 days.

Lycopodium 200C - Urine profuse during the night, tendency to retention with thick reddish sediment. Dose night and morning for 5 days.

Phosphorus 200C - Acute cases showing blood in urine, blood is diffused throughout the urine giving a brownish appearance. Dose night and morning for 3 days.

Nat Mur 200C - Chronic cases showing a pale urine of low specific gravity, there is usually salt retention leading to thirst and anemia. Dose night and morning for one week.

Urolithiasis - (Stones and Gravel)

This condition may arise from stasis of the urine. Seen more in males then females. Most stones in horses are found in the bladder. Various factors contribute especially the drinking of bore water but frequently the cause is not known.

Signs and Symptoms - Clinical signs depend on the location of the stone. There can be obvious difficulty in passing urine which can be scanty and blood stained. Affected horses frequently stretch out to urinate and may maintain this posture for variable periods before and after urination. Signs of pain include kicking at belly and looking around at flanks. The penis is usually relaxed during attempts to urinate. Urethral obstruction may also develop as the result of a trapped stone and is typically accompanied by restlessness, sweating, varying degrees of colic, and frequent attempts to urinate.

Herbal Treatment

Juliette de Bairacli Levy treats this condition with same treatment as for Nephritis. Couch grass should always be added to the Parsley or any of the other herbs given for the cure of Nephritis. Warm milk and molasses is highly beneficial for this complaint fortified with Slippery Elm Bark (one heaped tablespoon full to the quart) and nutmeg two teaspoon full. Also look at the herbs Cleavers, Bearberry, Gravel Root and Chaparral which are all Anti lithics. It is also wise to add some Demulcents to sooth the pain caused by gravel scraping its way down, some good ones for this system are Corn silk and Marshmallow. Use the Urinary Antiseptics if infection is present.

In gravel no grain foods should be fed for a period of one to 3 months. The diet should be hay, green feed and pulped roots. Of the cereals only bran is permitted and this should be feed daily with molasses in sufficient quantity to keep the bowels open. For this condition Pat Coleby gives a regular dose of cider vinegar which eventually breaks the stones down and stops them from reoccurring.

Homoeopathic Treatment

Lycopodium 200C - Hepatic symptoms with blood stained urine containing red sediment, the early stages of stone formation. Dose night and morning for 7 days.

Sarsaparilla 6C - Pain at the beginning and end of urination especially at the end, Urine contains gravelly deposits and is slimy. Dose 3 times daily for 3 days.

Urtica Urens 6X - Thickens the urine and removes the tendency to gravel formation by removing the basic salts that help form it, it will also increase the quantity of urine passed, there may be a skin rash, give one dose 3 times daily for 10 days.

Calc Phos 30C - A good constitutional remedy which will help regulate the calcium and phosphate metabolism and so prevent the formation of phosphates, it should be given as a routine remedy in young animals up till the age of one. One dose weekly for 8 weeks.

Mag Mur 6C - May help in preventing some forms of stones and may be given as a routine remedy if the urine shows suspicious deposits and there are other signs of stone formation.

Cystitis

Inflammation of the bladder can arise from a infection in some other part of the urinary system and a infection here can also travel up the ureters and infect the kidneys if not looked after. Cystitis can also arise as a result of stones and gravel damaging the delicate tissue and leaving it open for infection.

Signs and symptoms - Pulse and respiration may be increased, there is trembling of the hind legs accompanied by frequent straining to pass urine which may be so scanty as to pass drop by drop. There can be obvious pain. Urine Can be blood stained and may contain mucous. Paralysis of the muscular coat of the bladder is common in chronic cases shown by a inability to retain urine.

Herbal Treatment

The main herbs we use in cystitis are the Urinary Antiseptics with the best ones being Bearberry and Buchu. Cranberry is a good urinary antiseptic to as well as coating the pipe lines and preventing the adherence of bacteria. To the antiseptics we add Demulcents which sooth the irritated tissues with the best one for this condition being Corn Silk. You could add to the formula Gravel Root and Chaparral if you think the cause of the condition could be from urinary stones or gravel. Other herbs to consider are Yarrow, Agrimony, Cleavers, Damiana, Golden Rod, Plantain and Shepherds Purse. Pat Coleby thinks the cause of this condition is a lack of Vitamin A and says if the horse was regularly given a table spoon of Cod Liver Oil the condition would not occur. Also dose with Vitamin C to boost the immune system.

Homoeopathic Treatment.

Aconite 6C - In the early febrile involvement when pulse and respiration are increased. Dose every hour for 4 doses.

Cantharis 30C - Much straining and scanty amounts of bloody urine, there is hyper excitability and signs of sexual irritability. Dose night and morning in chronic cases for one week, in acute cases give one dose every hour for 4 doses.

Nux Vom 30C - When ineffectual urging is associated with digestive upsets. Dose 3 times daily for 2 days.

Dulcamara 30C - Catarrhal cystitis resulting from exposure to cold or damp, urine contains a thick mucus or purulent sediment. Dose 3 times daily for 3 days.

Causticum 30C - A useful remedy in the recurrent or chronic form and is especially adapted to the older animal. Follows well after Cantharis which may be needed if acute symptoms flare up in the chronic form.

Paralysis of the Bladder

In the early stages of paralysis the bladder remains full and dribbling of urine takes place. The bladder wall loses its muscle tone and the result is a build up to a chronic cystitis.

Homoeopathic Treatment

Gelsemium 200C - There is a profuse flow of pale urine which is expelled passively when the bladder becomes full. Dose night and morning for 5 days.

Conium 30C - When passage of urine starts and stops frequently. There is difficulty in expulsion. Condition may be accompanied by weakness of the back and hind limbs shown b y difficulty in rising. Dose 3 times daily for 4 days.

Herbal Overview Of The Urinary System

Most infections get to the kidneys via the blood for the kidneys are the main filter of the blood removing wastes and water. Other infections can start off as cystitis and travel up the ureter and infect the kidney that way so you must always consider both ways. Always ask yourself is the infection traveling from the kidneys down or the bladder up? If you think it is the kidney put a leash on the animal and walk them in tight circles one way and then the other. If the animal complains it is probably the kidney. Urinary antiseptics are good for this system whether for treating infection or preventing it as in cases of stones scraping the sides as they go down leaving a wound ripe for infection. Also think of Cranberry for this system as it coats the pipes and stops bacteria getting a foot hold literally.

Herbal Actions Of The Urinary System

Anti-biotic - Chaparral, Echinacea, Garlic, Myrrh, Pau D' Arco.

Anti-inflammatory - Helps the body to combat

inflammations.

Herbs - Cats Claw, Chaparral , Cleavers, Cranesbill, Eyebright, Ginger, Golden Rod, Guaiacum, Liquorice, Marshmallow, Pau D' Arco.

Anti-lithic - Prevent the formation of stones or gravel in the urinary system and helps the body to remove them.

Herbs - Bearberry, Corn Silk, Chaparral , Gravel Root, Horsetail.

Anti-microbial - Helps the body destroy or resist pathogenic micro-organisms.

Herbs - Echinacea, Garlic, Juniper, Myrrh,

Astringent - Contracts tissue which in turn reduces discharges, these herbs contain tannins.

Herbs - Agrimony, Cranesbill, Chaparral, Golden Rod, Horsetail, Shepherds Purse.

Cystitis - Agrimony, Bearberry, Buchu, Celery Seed, Corn Silk, Gravel Root, Golden Rod, Horsetail, Plantain,

Demulcent - Soothes and protects irritated or inflamed internal tissues.

Herbs - Bearberry, Corn Silk, Licorice, Marshmallow, Plantain, Slippery Elm.

Diuretic - Increases the secretion and elimination of urine.

Herbs - Agrimony Angelica, Bear Berry, Blue Flag, Burdock, Buchu, Broom, Coltsfoot, Chaparral, Corn Silk, Dandelion Leaves, Elder, Fumitory, Golden Rod, Guaiacum, Gravel Root, Hawthorn,

Horseradish, Horsetail, Juniper, Lime Blossom, Nettles, Pau D' Arco, Penny Royal, Plantain, Parsley, Shepherds Purse, Sarsaparilla, Yarrow.

Urinary Antiseptics - These herbs have a antiseptic action as they pass through the system.

Herbs - Angelica, Bearberry, Buchu, Corn Silk, Golden Rod, Shepherds Purse, Yarrow.

Notes

The Muscular Skeletal System

Myositis (muscle inflammation)

Inflammation of the muscle tissue may have its origin in a open wound or infection, or it may be the result of severe straining.

Signs and Symptoms - Local heat in the muscle is a early sign, followed by stiffness or lameness if leg muscles are involved. Febrile signs will accompany infectious conditions.

Herbal Treatment

If the cause is from bacterial infection then we would use our immune boosting herbs so as to start fighting the infection, these are Echinacea, Myrrh and Garlic. If inflammation is present treat with Anti-inflammatorys especially the ones that are pain killers - Willow bark and Devils Claw. If the inflammation was caused by injury try some of the First Aid remedies such as a compress of Arnica Lotion. Don't forget to look at the Homoeopathic First Aid remedies.

Homoeopathic Treatment.

Arnica 30C - Should always be given in the early inflammatory stage. Doses every 2 hours for 2 doses.

Apis 6C - Give if edema accompanies inflammation. Dose every 3 hours for 4 doses.

Rhus Tox 6C - Indicated when the animal gains relief from movement even though the initial movement is painful, symptoms may be more on the left side of the body then the right, indicated when severe wetting or prolong dampness is associated with the onset of the symptoms.

Bryonia 30C - Movement is resented when Bryonia is indicated. The animal will seek to lie on the affected muscles and pressure on them gives ease, warmth is usually useful also.

Hepar Sulph 30C - Infection from a open scratch or wound. Dose 3 times daily for 3 days.

Osteoarthritis

Degenerative joint disease of a non-inflammatory origin where the articular cartilages become eroded and bony exostoses occur at the margin of the joints. Although age plays a part there can be other causes such as systemic or metabolic disturbances. Progressive mild inflammation in the joint over a period of time is more likely to produce osteoarthritis than any other predisposing factor. Osteoarthritis particularly affects the load bearing bones of the body. Being overweight adds to the wear and tear of the joints. Once the cartilage degenerates the cushioning effect is lost within the joint and the joint capsule now becomes involved and the situation becomes worse.

Signs and Symptoms - Lameness is the main sign and it could involve several joints. The articular surfaces of the cervical vertebrae are sometimes affected in the horse. This may cause pain and difficulty of movement. A unwillingness to use the affected part results in muscular wasting of the area, later signs include thickening of the joint, the worst affected limb may be held in a flexed manner. Involvement of the stifle joint may lead to a fracture to the head of the tibia causing complete recumbency. When the hip joint is effected reduction of the head of the femur takes place.

Herbal Treatment

Nutrition wise for the early stages you can give calcium, Vitamin D, magnesium, manganese and boron which is probably the most important as this is the mineral that hardens the surface of bones and is usual deficient in soils where arthritis is common, you should be able to find all of these together in a good calcium formula. This formula especially with the boron should stop the condition from getting worse. Glucosamine and Chondroitin Sulphate can help stimulate the rebuilding of cartilage and help in the early stages of arthritis along with having a anti-inflammatory action.

Arthritis with lots of pain and inflammation needs the use of the Anti-Inflammatory herbs, good ones to use for this condition are Meadowsweet, Devils Claw and Willow bark as these act as good pain killers as well. Other herbs to use are the Alteratives which clean out the area and the system some good ones are Burdock, Garlic, Sarsaparilla and Chaparral which has a antioxidant action as well. Diuretic herbs are also used for this condition as they help to remove the metabolic waste and toxins which usually result from the constant inflammation and help the kidneys flush this waste out, some good ones are Celery seed (the acid remover), Juniper (these two are best used together) and Dandelion leaf. Other herbs to look at for arthritis are Black Cohosh, Cats Claw, Guaiacum, Nettles, Wild yam and Yellow dock. Add Liquorice to the formula at about 10% as this will help in the assimilation of the formula into the body and add a anti-inflammatory and demulcent action.

Below is a another Arthritis Formula

Yucca - root powder 2 cups

Wild Yam - root powder 2 cups

Chaparral - leaves 1 cup

Comfrey - root 2 cups

Sarsaparilla - root 1 cup

Horsetail - plant powder quarter cup. (do not use this continuously see warning a back of book)

Add 2 cups of boiling water to 4 tablespoons of the mixed herb and let steep for 20 minutes, mix with feed twice daily.

Homoeopathic Treatment

Not an easy condition to treat. Start treatment as early as possible so as to slow down deterioration. Useful remedies for the early inflammatory stages are.

Rhus Tox 6C - This remedy is indicated when the animal's symptoms are eased after a short period of movement. There may be initial stiffness on first moving.

Bryonia 6C - The indications for this remedy are the opposite of the above, the animal prefers to remain still and any movement causes distress and sometimes acute pain evidenced by the animal crying out.

Calc Flour 30C - May be needed in the latter stages once the exostoses and joint swellings develop. The carpus is the main joint affected when this remedy is indicated. There may be accompanying cystic tumors around the joint.

Rhus Tox 1M - This can be given in the latter stages to help with the symptoms of pain when the animal moves.

Rheumatism

Herbal Treatment

The way Juliette de Bairacli Levy treats this condition is by giving for the diet give good hay and a generous ration of oats and bran. Chopped Celery plant stems and leaves also water-cress, Parsley - including the roots and Comfrey should be included with the oats when available plus a little molasses, and the horse should get at least 2 handfuls of nettles (lightly boiled for 2 minutes only) daily. Dock, Juniper bark, Burdock and Willow bark are all proved excellent and handfuls of Primrose flowers mixed in bran mashes. (you could consider giving primrose or fish oil tablets) A Gypsy name for rheumatism in horses is Flying Lameness on account of the frequent shifting from one area of the body to another. Local relief should not be considered a cure. The whole body must be rendered pain free for a period of months before a cure can be sure. A brew of rosemary and salt

(salt alkalizes the acid) has proved excellent. To this I would add a dose of Cod Liver oil once a week for its vitamin A which has a action on the mucous membranes. Look at the Anti-Rheumatic herbs in the Herbal Actions List.

Homoeopathic Treatment

Use the remedies listed under Osteoarthritis with the addition of Aconite and Formica.

Arthritis Due To Infection

This is caused by pyogenic bacteria getting in the joint mainly from injury the main organisms are Streptococci and Staphylococci. In new born foals a common cause is the bacteria traveling up the umbilical cord wound.

Signs and Symptoms - There may be a initial temperature rise and febrile signs may develop. The affected joint becomes enlarged and swollen, stiff, tense and hot due to inflammation. Pain is obvious by the onset of severe lameness. Examination may reveal the presence of punctures on the skin and the appearance of a purulent exudate. The hock, stifle and carpus are the joints chiefly affected while in foal involvement of several joints is common. This condition is serious and could lead to permanent damage if action is not taken fast.

Note - Brucellosis is a disease which has now become recognized as a cause of bacterial arthritis in the horse.

Herbal Treatment

For this condition think of our infection fighting herbs such as Echinacea, Garlic and Myrrh. If the skin is broken and you think the infection got in this way apply a lotion of Calendula and St Johns Wort to the area. To our infection fighting herbs you can add some of the Anti Inflammatorys, Alteratives and Diuretics that are mentioned in Osteo Arthritis. Add Liquorice to the formula at about 10% as this will help in the assimilation of the formula into the body. If the condition is serious you may need professional help to lance , drain and wash out the wound.

Homoeopathic Treatment

Aconitum 30C - This should be given as soon as possible in the early febrile stage.

Ferrum Phos 6C - This also is a good remedy for the initial feverish stage more often indicated when throat symptoms accompany the invasive process.

Belladonna 30C - Indicated when the patient presents a excitable picture with dilated pupils, throbbing arteries and a hot skin.

Bryonia 6C - Symptoms worse for movement, relief from pain on pressure over the joint and a possible involvement with the respiratory tract. The joint is usually extremely hard and tense.

Apis Mel 6C - If the synovial sheaf of the joint becomes edematous indicated by swelling this remedy may help. The patient is made worse by heat in any form and does not drink much.

Ledum 6C - The remedy of choice if the arthritis has

been caused by the penetration of a sharp object giving rise to a puncture wound.

Iodum 6C - This is a remedy which sometimes gives good results in the less acute case especially when the joint pains are worse at night. The patient is often thin with a voracious appetite and the skin is dry and withered looking.

Rhus Tox 6C - The indications for this remedy are relief from movement although there may be initial stiffness on rising. There may be accompanying skin symptoms of a vesicular itchy nature.

Silica 30C - This remedy is indicated in the more chronic case. There may be involvement of neighboring lymphatic glands showing cold abscesses.

Bursitis

Bursa is the term generally employed to include all synovial sacs and refers to the true bursa situated between the tendon and the bone or between two tendons and also includes joint capsules and synovial sheath. Damage to the bursa of the joint due to overweight is a common contributory factor as is also irritation of the part by repeated contact with the ground if the animal is inclined to rest more than usual. The pain in acute bursitis may be relieved by the application of cold packs and in bad cases aspiration of the contents. Treatment of chronic bursitis is surgical. In infected bursitis, systemic antibiotics as well as local drainage may be required.

Signs and Symptoms - The acute form shows swelling, heat and pain evidenced by lameness. Effusion into the bursa occurs and accounts in part to the increase of size. When bursitis is chronic fibrotic changes take place leading to the formation of a solid lump in the affected area. This may eventually ulcerate leading to secondary infection.

Herbal Treatment

Liniments made from essential oils in a base of olive oil can be applied to the area, Cayenne and Ginger would increase the circulation to the area while Wintergreen would act as a good pain killer along with Peppermint. Other essential oils are St Johns Wort, Lavender and Rosemary. If the condition is becoming chronic treat with Anti Inflammatory herbs. If the condition is infected treat with the Antibacterial immune boosting herbs with Echinacea being the best for blood borne bacteria. Cold packs can also help relieve the pain and swelling.

Homoeopathic Treatment

Apis Mel 30C - Useful in the early inflammatory stage where effusion is taking place and the joint is extremely tender to touch, The animal may lick and gnaw at the joint because of itching and irritation. Patient shows a intolerance to heat and touch. Apis is always good for sharp pains and swellings.

Bryonia 6C - Indicated when the joint is enlarged and pressure over the area brings relief as does the application of cold compresses. The animal resents movement and prefers to lie on the effected joint.

Rhus Tox 6C - If surrounding ligaments and tendons are involved to any great extent this remedy will be needed, movement limbers up the animal which is in need of Rhus Tox.

Calc Flour 30C - This is a good general tissue remedy and has a beneficial effect on the development of cysts, cystic tumors and fibrous swellings.

Hepar Sulphuris 200C - Purulent bursitis, Extreme tenderness and sensitivity to touch. Dose every 3 hours for 4 doses.

Silica 30C - This is another good long term remedy which will help dissolve any associated scar and fibrous tissue. It will be beneficial if surface ulceration occurs leading to secondary infection.

Laminitis

This is a painful condition where circulatory changes cause inflammation and congestion to the sensitive laminae of the feet. This condition is not well understood but it is believed there is a rise in blood pressure that increases pressure to the feet which in turn mucks up the circulation of the feet causing swelling and inflammation. This inflammation restricts blood, oxygen and nutrient supply then forces the pedal bone down close to the surface causing sensitivity and pain. The causes seem to be from overweight, wrong diet, and impact injury from hard surfaces. There are acute and chronic forms of this condition.

Signs and Symptoms - If the front feet are

effected sometimes the animal stands with the rear feet kind of close to the middle of the body so as to take the weight off the front and on the affected area the horse tries to stand on the heels. There is obvious pain with the horse moving from one foot to another. Usually, heat is apparent in the whole hoof, especially near the coronary band. An exaggerated and bounding pulse can be felt and may be visible in the digital arteries. Pain can cause muscular trembling, and a fairly uniform tenderness can be detected when pressure is applied to the feet. The pedal bone may rotate during or after the acute stage if treatment is not given rapidly.

The animal doesn't want to move and the feet are raised with great difficulty. In very severe case a blood-stained exudate may seep from the coronary bands. (call a vet immediately). Chronic laminitis is characterized by changes in the shape of the hoof and the bands around it and usually follows one or more attacks of the acute form.

Herbal Treatment

For the acute attack it is best to get a vet as this is a painful and dangerous condition. I shall start off with the treatment used in the past but bear in mind that this condition was not common in the past as most horses had fairly natural diets so this gives us our main clue in prevention.

Juliette de Bairacli Levy treats this condition by removing the shoes and poulticing the feet with hot bran and salt, a teacup of salt to a quart of bran.

Personally I would leave the shoes on but still poultice as the salt would draw some of the internal excess fluid out. Another old favorite is a turnip poultice, 4 boiled and mashed to each leg kept warm and wet. As soon as the temperature is normal again walk on soft grass for 30 minutes 3 times daily.

I would treat this condition by changing the diet and especially reducing the protein in the diet. Try to make it a more natural one. Start treatment by fasting the animal. The herb I would start with is Hawthorn so as to normalize the blood pressure and as I think this condition has a lot to do with the liver I would give Milk Thistle which would start by taking the load off the liver and in turn decrease venous congestion which with the Hawthorn may normalize the circulation. Look at the chapter on the circulatory system for more herbs. I would also use the salt poultice above.

Homoeopathic Treatment

Aconite 30C - Give as soon as symptoms begin as this will help with the anxiety and regulate pulse and respiration. Dose every 30 minutes for 6 doses.

Belladonna 1M - Full bounding pulse, throbbing arteries, heat and sweating and there may be irritability. Dose every 30 minutes for 6 doses.

Nux Vom 1M - Systemic Congestion, irritable, does not want to be touched. Dose every 2 hours for 4 doses.

Calc Flour 30C - May promote a return to normal structure in the chronic case. (see the Cell Salts or

Tissue Salts)

Bone Injuries and Fractures

Herbal Treatment

The main remedy here is comfrey or to use its old fashioned name knitbone. This is good to use internally and on the injured area when the cast is removed as it will help to strengthen the mend. For areas that do not have casts on or for fine fractures Comfrey is ideal and will speed up the healing process. Comfrey has a chemical in it that speeds up cell division it is also astringent and demulcent which gives it soothing and protecting qualities and has been used for hundreds of years in the healing of bones and wounds. Some people grow this herb and then turn it into liquid manure as it is one of the most mineral rich herbs around.

Treatment

Apply cream to affected area regularly, if you grow Comfrey in your garden you can make a poultice out of the leaves and apply it to the affected area.

Homoeopathic Treatment

Follow normal first aid procedures, if the bone is obviously broken it is best to call a vet. If you do have to move the patient make sure the injured limb is supported or a sharp piece of bone may cut a internal artery. Most bone injuries need x-rays to determine the extent of the damage.

Remedies with leading symptoms

Arnica 6 to 30C - Can be given straight away for the shock and will help ease the pain from the bruising and swelling.

Ledum 6 to 30C - Take after arnica 4 hourly or 3 times a day to assist in the absorption of the extravasation of blood after a fracture so as to reduce the swelling which may take up to 3 to 4 days. (helps to absorb the internal bleeding after a fracture)

After the bones have been set properly use these two remedies.

Calc Phos 6X - Helps in nutrition especially of the bones and promotes the knitting together of the bones. Helps fractures heal much faster. Can be used in alternation with Symphytum. Calc Phos is what is known as a Biochemic Tissue Salt and can be brought in most chemists.

Symphytum 6 to 30C - More commonly known as comfrey or knitbone or bone set. The name says it all. Promotes fast healing of bones, use with Calc Phos 6X. Take both 3 times daily till recovered.

Sprains and Strains

Herbal Treatment

Severe sprains usually need a supporting bandage and a medical checkup to see if there has been any other damage. A lot of damage and trauma can be prevented if the injured area was put under cold water or ice immediately after the injury the quicker the less the damage. For a bad sprain I would use lots of Arnica cream to start with and at night apply Arnica and Comfrey mixed creams along with a support bandage for the area so as to keep the cream there and also for the extra heat to the area that would create. If you grow Comfrey in your garden then you could put on a Comfrey poultice at night. Ginger is another herb that could be used in a poultice at night.

Treatment

Cold water or ice immediately

Arnica Cream (do not apply on open wounds)

Comfrey Cream mixed with arnica cream overnight

Ginger poultice overnight.

Comfrey poultice overnight.

Calendula - Healing and soothing.

Homoeopathic Treatment

Joint problems due to twisting, wrenching or over use. A sprain is damaged tendons or ligaments while a strain happens when the connecting tissues around a joint are over stretched. Use your normal first aid procedures and support the joint with supporting bandage and give the appropriate remedies with the first one being Arnica. If there is no sign of improvement in 24 to 36 hours get checked for a fracture.

Arnica 6 to 30C - For the shock and bruised sore pains. Arnica cream can also be applied as long as the skin is not broken.

Bellis Perennis 6 to 30C - Deeper acting then arnica, intense soreness of the muscles, where swellings and lumps remain after the injury.

Ledum 6 to 30C - Injuries where the swollen part is cold or numb, sometimes looks purple and puffy, feels better for cold applications.

Ruta 6 to 30C - If the bones inside or near the joint feel bruised

Herbal Overview Of The Muscular Skeletal System

For bruising think about Arnica in a lotion and use the Homoeopathic dose internally, for broken bones think about Comfrey as its old name is knit bone. For arthritis and rheumatism use your Anti Rheumatics, Anti Inflammatorys, and Analgesics but also think of Celery Seed as this is called the acid remover and another herb to think of is Meadowsweet as this herb is called the acid balancer. It is usually the high acid in the system that irritates the joints and starts the inflammation so these 2 herbs could remove the cause for the condition; also consider diet as a diet high in protein will create a lot of acid waste. For blood borne bacterial infections think of the Alteratives (blood cleansers) and Anti Bacterials especially our main ones Garlic and Echinacea. If there is damage to the joints use a nutritional supplement with these 3 together - Glucosamine Sulphate, Chondroitin and MSM as these together will help rebuild the joints.

Herbal Actions For The Muscular Skeletal System

Alterative - Herbs that gradually restore proper function to the body, they increase health and vitality. They were once known as the blood cleansers.
Herbs - Black Cohosh, Blue Flag, Burdock,

Chaparral, Echinacea, Garlic, Nettles, Pau D'Arco ,Sarsaparilla, Yellow Dock.

Analgesic - Herbs that reduce pain.

Herbs - Black Cohosh, Chamomile, Hops, Meadowsweet, Pau D'Arco, Peppermint, Skullcap, St Johns Wort, Valerian.

Anti-biotic - Chaparral, Echinacea, Garlic, Myrrh, Pau D' Arco.

Antispasmodic - Prevents or eases spasms and cramps.

Herbs - Angelica, Black Cohosh, Chamomile, Skullcap, St johns Wort, Valerian.

Anti-inflammatory - Helps the body to combat inflammations.

Herbs - Cats Claw, Devils Claw, Chaparral , Feverfew, Ginger, Guaiacum, Liquorice, Meadowsweet, Pau D' Arco, Sarsaparilla, St Johns Wort, Willow Bark.

Anti-viral - Astragalus, Cats claw, Echinacea, Garlic, Myrrh?, St Johns Wort, Pau D'Arco.

Anti-Rheumatic - Angelica, Burdock, Black Cohosh, Chaparral, Cats Claw, Celery Seed, Dandelion, Garlic, Guaiacum, Nettles, Willow Bark, Yellow Dock.

Rubefacient - Causes a gentle local irritation to the skin which stimulates the capillaries to open increasing the blood flow.

Herbs - Cayenne, Garlic, Ginger, Horseradish, Nettles, Peppermint Oil, Rosemary Oil, Rue.

Skin And Coat Problems

Dermatitis

This term implies an inflammation of the skin. It may be Bacterial or Viral in origin but a allergic form is more common in the horse.

Signs and Symptoms - Erythema (redness) is the first sign, vesicular lesions may then occur followed by edema in severe cases. This condition can look similar to Eczema but may be more of an allergic type of reaction then true Eczema.

Herbal Treatment

For a true dermatitis the best cure is to remove the cause and the same goes if the condition is a response to a allergic reaction. See the herbal section for Eczema especially the herbs that are used for external treatment.

Homoeopathic Treatment

Arsenic Alb 1M - Dry Dermatitis. Thirst, restless, worse after midnight. Dose daily for ten days.

Rhus Tox 1M - Vesicles may form in the early erythematous stage and can be itchy, stiffness in joints which get better with movement. Dose 3 times daily for 2 days.

Antimonium Tart 30 - Early stages of vesicular formation. Respiratory symptoms accompany this condition. Dose night and morning for 3 days.

Thuja 200C - Chronic state showing thickening of the skin. Dose once a day for 2 weeks.

Apis 6C - Shiny liquid filled swellings that pit under

pressure and are hot and tender, could be mainly on the abdomen. Dose 2 hourly for 4 doses.

Urtica Urens 6C - Where there is acute irritation, small red weals which aggravate, hot and itchy with a tendency to edema. Dose 3 times daily for 3 days.

Eczema

This term covers skin complaints which produce a inflammation of epidermal cells. It can arise from internal or external factors. It may be environmental in origin or from excessive sweating or repeated wetting or it could be a genetic factor.

Signs and Symptoms - The initial lesion is raw looking, followed by weeping of the skin. Itching is usually intense and the hair may come out of the affected area. Eczema is a general term used for any inflammatory process involving the skin marked by redness, itching, papules and vesicles, weeping, oozing, crusting and later by scaling and often pigmentation.

Herbal Treatment

If the condition is true Eczema (find family history) then the problem will be hard to get rid of as Eczema is usually a very deep seated disease. Herbally you would use the deep acting Alterative herbs which would slowly deeply cleanse the body and blood hopefully removing the seat of the problem.

Some Alterative herbs are Blue Flag, Burdock, Garlic, Fumitory, Nettles and Sarsaparilla with Burdock and Sarsaparilla being the best to start with. Also ensure that there are Essential Fatty Acids in the diet as these will help to tone down the inflammatory process. Consider also the Anti-Inflammatory actions and the Emollient Actions. For this condition Pat Coleby gives extra zinc which can be given in the form of seaweed meal or zinc sulphate. She says seaweed meal works the best.

Externally given as a lotion or ointment consider the following which can be mixed. Chickweed is good for the itching and helps with the healing especially if mixed with Calendula. Consider also Burdock, Neem and Witch hazel.

Homoeopathic Treatment

Sulphur 30C - Lesions are red and look wet, itching is intense, worse for warmth. Dose night and morning for 5 days.

Arsenic Alb 1M - Dry eczema, animal is thirsty and seeks warmth, symptoms worse after midnight, animal becomes more restless. Dose once daily for 2 weeks.

Rhus Tox 1M - Condition is vesicular and itchy, stiffness in joints which get better with movement. Dose daily for 5 days.

Antimonium Crud 6C - Eczema accompanied by stomach upsets, worse at night. Dose night and morning for 3 days.

Anacardium 200C - Nervousness, skin reddish and very itchy with vesicular eruption. Dose night and morning for 5 days.

Petroleum 200C - Blistery eruptions with tendency to

suppuration of cracked skin which bleeds easily, skin usually dry. Dose night and morning for 1 week.

Psorinum 30C - Dry lusterless skin with severe itching, the associated lymph glands are swollen. Sometimes a oily skin has ulceration which heals slowly. A unpleasant smell accompanies the eczema. Dose night and morning for 1 week.

Graphites 6C - Discharge of sticky honey colored fluid, skin is usually dry and itchy, hairs fall out. Dose 3 times daily for 3 days.

Cantharis 200C - Severe vesicular eczema, symptoms worse in cold dry conditions and better in warm damp conditions.

Mange - Leg Mange

Caused by the mite Chorioptes equi . The signs subside in summer but recur with the return of cold weather. Ensure that the diet is adequate and the horse is clean and in good condition as this is the best way to prevent the problem.

Signs and Symptoms - Leg mange effects the lower limbs of draught type horses but in heaver infestations can extend to the upper limbs, armpits and groin. The mites cause extensive irritation as they bite and feed. The skin becomes moist with a bloody exudate. Affected horses repeatedly stamp their feet when being examined. At the beginning of mange there is little or nothing to be seen only that the animal rubs themselves, but after a time numerous small pimples appear out of which a watery fluid oozes and on exposure to air dries and forms a scab on which the hair stands erect. If the disease is allowed to go on unchecked ulcers are frequently produced. This condition is very contagious and you will have to check the rest of the animals so as to see if it has spread and maybe find where it came from.

Herbal Treatment

A horse with mange requires a preliminary all over washing with lots of soap and warm water to which a little soda has been added followed by a thorough cleansing with a hose before any curative treatment can be applied. A scurfy mane and tail can be cleansed by rubbing briskly with a warm strong brew of Rosemary herb and then massaging well with a little castor oil which stimulates long and supple hair growth. Some insecticide herbs are Neem, Aniseed, Garlic and Rosemary. Use the external herbs mentioned in eczema for healing. The mentioned herbs can be mixed in a spray bottle and sprayed on. Below is a formula for dogs using Essential Oils.

Mange Treatment Blend

15ml base oil of hazel nut or sweet almond oil

5 drops Lavender

7 drops Niaouli

1 drop Helichrysum

2 drops Sweet Marjoram

After bathing the dog 2 to 4 drops of the blend should be applied to the affected areas twice a day for at least 2 weeks. Observe for a week and repeat if necessary.

Homoeopathic Treatment

Sulphur 30C - Lesions are red and look wet, itching is intense, worse for warmth. Dose night and morning for 5 days.

Arsenic Alb 30C - If the hair falls off and the skin becomes loose and flabby or if there are ulcers with hard red edges, dry eczema, animal is thirsty and seeks warmth, symptoms worse after midnight, animal becomes more restless. Dose once daily for 2 weeks.

Sepia 30C - If the effected parts are tender and the animal shrinks when touched or if there are white looking blisters filled with a watery fluid. Dose 3 times a day.

Rhus Tox 30C- Condition is vesicular and itchy, stiffness in joints which get better with movement. Dose 3 times daily.

Ringworm

Ringworm lesions in the horse may be superficial or deep with the former being the more common. This condition is a fungal infection that is highly contagious between animals and can be passed on by sharing of saddles and harnesses. Most infections are seen in young horses during the humid months of the year.

Signs and Symptoms - Irritation and itching may first occur with the lesions developing initially on the rump and trunk before spreading to other parts. The

Ringworm fungus causes loss of hair in circular patches that progressively get larger. Single centers of hair loss are usually up to 3 centimeters across and can join together to produce large areas. Most are scaly and dry but can be moist if the hair has matted together and there is a secondary infection.

Herbal Treatment

Ringworm is a fungal infection which usually attacks when the immune system is weakened by stress or exhaustion. Fungi thrive in damp, dark and confined places. If you think the immune system is run down you can give Echinacea, zinc, and vitamin C and you might as well give Garlic as this has a anti-fungal action. Externally treatment can be a lotion of Calendula 1 to 5 in strength for cleaning the area and around it. Stronger anti-fungals may be necessary as this can sometimes be a very stubborn condition to get rid of. Garlic is a stronger anti-fungal and you can use this externally and internally at the same time. Another strong anti-fungal we have is Tea Tree oil which can be put on neat to the infected area. Pau D Arco is a good herb to think of for this condition as it is a Immune Booster and Anti-Fungal together. For this condition Pat Coleby says the cause is a sulphur deficiency. A wash of 20% of copper sulphate in water scrubbed well in will kill the infection. She says for tender areas use cider vinegar alone.

Treatment

Raise immunity.

Calendula lotion 1 to 5 strength on and around the

affected area. (can mix with garlic)

Tea tree oil - Strong anti-fungal dab on to the affected area neat.

Garlic externally On effected area and latter if problem is not resolving take internally.

Raw lemon Juice applied twice daily.

Other herbs to look at are Burdock, Elder, Sarsaparilla, Myrrh and Rue.

Homoeopathic Treatment

Bacillinum 200C - 2 doses at two week intervals with sepia 6C.

Tellurium 30C - Twice a day for one week especially when lesions tend to be equally distributed on either side of the body.

Chrysarobinum 6C - 3 times a day for 5 days, when the disease has progressed to the crusty stage.

Note - Animals that are susceptible to ringworms are usually deficient in copper.

Acne

Infection of hair follicles by bacteria. This seems to be a mixture of many factors with a lot of them having to do with sebum which is the oil produced in the hair follicles which increases production due to the increased hormones in puberty . This condition can also occur in pressure areas.

Signs and Symptoms - Lesions commence as nodules quickly becoming pustular and spreading to other neighboring follicles.

Herbal Treatment.

1. Make a poultice of slippery elm as this draws out the impurities and opens the pores.
2. Calendula lotion in a 1 to 20 mix helps to regulate the skins production of oil as well as being disinfecting and healing. You can use the comfrey cream as well to prevent scaring if needed.

Another Effective Method

1. Tea Tree oil dabbed on effected area frequently.
2. Give the Tissue Salt Calc Sulph (chemist or health shops will have it) Follow directions on the label.

Homoeopathic treatment

Hepar Sulphuris 200C - This remedy has a wide range of action and should be considered in any suppurative process showing extreme sensitivity to touch indicating acute pain. Low potencies of this remedy promote suppuration while high potencies (200 plus) may abort the purulent process and promote resolution.

Sulphur Iodatum 6C - Associated eczema with reddening of the skin. Dose night and morning for one week.

Arsenicum Alb 1M - When the skin is dry and itchy, the animal is restless and thirsty. Dose daily for 10 days.

Ledum 6C - Acne associated with facial eczema. Itching made worse by warmth. Dose night and morning for 1 week.

Antimonium Crudum 6C - Warty excrescences and dry skin. Hard scabs appear over pustules. Dose night and morning for 5 days.

Queensland Itch

The cause of this condition is a allergy to the bite of the sand fly. To protect against flies always let the horse keep its full and natural length of the mane and tail with which it swishes away the flies.

Signs and Symptoms - When the horse is bitten by the sand fly small lumps develop in the skin. Because the lumps are intensely itchy the horse rubs itself causing loss of hair. Serum oozes from the skin and scabs form. In chronic cases the skin becomes thickened and corrugated especially along the flank, neck, buttocks and tail. Other diseases that can look similar include ring worm, tail itch, stable and buffalo fly bites and rain scald.

Herbal Treatment

For the initial itching after being bitten by sand flies mix some Baking Soda with water and paint this solution onto the affected area and this should bring some relief always consider doing this first as it draws the toxins out relieving the itch. For itchy areas where the hair has fallen out and the skin is becoming damaged use a lotion of Calendula and Chickweed so as to relieve the itching and encourage tissue healing. The next I copy from a old Herbal on Horses and you will have to experiment for yourself. Treat areas where flies gather by applying a light rub of waste motor oil (sump oil) add a few drops of Eucalyptus oil to each pint for extra good effect.

Avoid the eyes. Rub strong wine vinegar morning and night into the hoofs and up to the fetlocks as this penetrates the body and discourages flies and mosquitoes.

Saddle Sores

The area of riding horses that is under saddle, or the shoulder area of those driven in harness, is frequently the site of injuries to the skin and deeper soft and bony tissues. These injuries are usually the result of friction from bad fitting saddles or back pads. This is also true for sore shoulders, necks and breasts which are mostly the results of dirty, badly fitting shoulder or breast collars. When the skin and underlying tissues are damaged more seriously or are continuously damaged abscesses may develop. The injury will keep on becoming more severe until the cause is removed so start here. Remember that it is important to keep the collar and saddle clean along with the rest of the harness.

Signs and Symptoms - Affected areas show hair loss and are swollen, warm, and painful. The serous or purulent exudate dries and forms crusts. The hair follicles may be inflamed or there may be boils in the areas rubbed. Advanced lesions are termed "galls and are characterized by warm, fluctuating, painful swellings from which purulent and fluid can be aspirated.

Herbal Treatment

The main treatment is to remove the cause. Look

under the headings bruises, boils and wounds and choose your appropriate treatment.

Bruises

Bruises are usually impact injuries caused by blows or falls and usually heal fairly fast. When there has been substantial bruising or a high enough impact to cause shock consider using the remedies below. Bruises are caused from blood vessels that have ruptured under the skin as a result of trauma, as the blood from the broken vessels is slowly absorbed the color slowly disappears.

Herbal Treatment

Arnica is the main remedy that is used for bruising mainly as a lotion or a cream but it must not be used where the skin is broken. If used on broken skin it will cause a bad reaction. Arnica is good for the bruised like pain in limbs and joints which have been over used or sprained as well as your everyday type of bruises. Cold compresses can bring relief as well.

For bruises where there are open wounds such as cuts and grazes use St Johns Wort and Calendula together in a lotion and later you could mix the creams together and apply as healing resumes.

Homoeopathic Treatment

Arnica 6 to 30C - For bruised soft tissues, muscles and connective tissue. Rapidly aids in the absorption of effused blood. The swelling which usually accompanies bruising reduces fairly quickly but if there is little reaction use **Ledum**. Arnica cream can be used on the external area of the wound.

Caution - Arnica must not be used on or near broken skin only use Calendula or Hypericm cream on wounds.

Bellis Perennis 6 to 30C - Follows after and is similar to arnica but is used for the deeper internal bruising while arnica is more external. Good for trauma and wounds of the pelvic and abdominal organs.

Ledum 6 to 30C - Helps in blood reabsorbing, may be needed if swelling remains after taking arnica. Affected parts are cold and worse for warmth.

Hypericum 6 to 30C - For bruised nerves, use where there is sharp shooting pains in punctured or penetrating wounds, for bruises of nerve rich areas such as the fingers, tail bone, lips and nose. Hypercal cream can be applied to the site externally.

Ruta 6 to 30C - Bruises of the bone or the bone covering the periosteum, good for shin bone injuries.

Note - Hypercal cream can be used externally on bruises where the skin is broken as arnica cream or lotion cannot be used on broken skin.

Abscesses and Boils

These are typically caused by a bacterial infection usually starting in a hair follicle. The first stage is characterized by a painful red swelling after which pus begins to form, this will usually discharge itself in a few days. Do not squeeze as this usually causes internal damage and a spread of the wound and infection.

Herbal Treatment

For lots of boils or recurring boils think of a course of Echinacea and Garlic maybe followed by Burdock so as to clean up the blood. Hot poultices are very effective at drawing the core out of boils so here we shall use a hot poultice of Slippery Elm (half a tea spoon full) with about 4 drops of Castor Oil which is also good at drawing out unwanted matter, mix this with a bit of boiling water to form a hot paste. Apply to the area and leave on for 20 minutes and repeat several times till suppuration occurs. After suppuration you can mix together a bit of Calendula and Comfrey creams and apply them to the area. These two herbs working together will speed up the healing time, disinfect and reduce or prevent scaring.

Homoeopathic Treatment

A boil is a infected, reddened, swollen area of the skin usually in a hair follicle or some other pit in the skin. Boils can be very painful while they develop until they come to a head and burst.

Remedies with leading symptoms

Hypericum Lotion - Make at a strength of 1 to 25 parts water ,soak a compress and apply reasonably wet to the affected area. Take Tarantula at the time.

Hepar Sulph 6C - To ripen a slow forming boil or abscess.

Silica 6C- For more advanced boils to encourage them to discharge, for foul smelling discharges or incomplete discharges.

Tarantula cubenis 6C - For painful hard feeling boils

that develop rapidly after a slow start especially on the back of the neck or on boils where the skin turns red blue or purple. Give this remedy 3 or 4 times daily along with a Hypericum compress taped over the area.

Burns

If you live in countries like Australia then fire is common and you will have to deal with it at least once in your life, with me it was at night and the fire followed the long grass of the fence line to the back of the stable and tried to set that alight to while I was frantically trying to get the nervous horses out. Get all burns under cold water immediately; always remember that burns keep on burning inwards for about 15 seconds after the heat source is removed. On first degree burns the skin becomes red only. 2nd degree the burn begins to destroy living tissue, blisters develop, 3rd degree the burns are deep and involve all layers of the skin, these are life threatening depending on the size of the area mainly through the loss of fluids and the risk of infections.

Herbal Treatment

For minor burns and scolds Aloe Vera gel straight from the plants leaf can give quick relief and speed up the healing. In herbalism we use the Astringents for burns (with the exception being for burns that cover a very large area) as the tannins in the herbs will seal and protect the burned surface and they also have a antibiotic action. Deep burns always require prompt medical attention. As the burns begin to heal you can use a mixture of Calendula and St Johns Wort cream on the healing edges.

Aloe Vera - Apply to burn straight from the plant.

Witch Hazel - Use as a lotion at about 1 to 20 strength and apply to the burn, this herb is a strong astringent and should seal and protect the surface.

Once the healing has begun you can continue applying Aloe vera especially if there is still pain. Another good herb for the pain is St Johns Wort which you could apply as a lotion. The best way to do this is from a spray bottle that gives off a fine mist.

Homoeopathic Treatment

Remedies with leading symptoms.

Calendula Cream - Use this on the edges of the burn as the burn heals.

Causticum 6 to 30C - For 2nd degree burns taken as needed for the pain with Hypericum lotion used externally on the burn and calendula cream on the edges.

Cantharis 6 to 30C - For 3rd degree burns taken as needed. This time wait for the healing to begin before using Hypericum and calendula as mentioned with Causticum.

Hypericum - To be used as a lotion 20 drops of tincture to 1 cup of water. (soothes the pain).

Urtica Urens 6 to 30C - For first degree burns taken as needed internally for the pain with Hypericum lotion used externally.

Cuts and Wounds

Herbal Treatment

The first consideration is to stop the bleeding, rule out any deeper internal damage and clean and disinfect the wound. To stop the bleeding refer to bleeding section. Calendula is one of the main lotions used for cleaning wounds as it is gentle, soothing, healing and anti-microbial so it kills the germs as well. Calendula has a tendency of sometimes welding the skin together (handy for closing knife like cuts) this is more noticeable on wounds with clean cut edges. Because of this tendency it is very important to make sure that all wounds are very clean and no dirt remains inside. I use Hypericum (St Johns Wort) lotion on wounds that are in very nerve rich areas, a good example is crush injuries to the lips as we all know how painful and sensitive a wound is to this area. As well as being used for nerve damage Hypericm is also astringent so it will help in stopping the bleeding and its anti-inflammatory action should help to reduce the swelling, this herb is also used to prevent tetanus. I usually get a separate bottle and fill it up with half Hypericum and half Calendula tincture and call this bottle Hypercal. I use this bottle for making my lotions for wounds on nervy areas. One of the leading symptoms for Hypericum is shooting pains along the nerve path from the injured area.

Treatment

1. Deal with bleeding and clean wound under running tap or hose water if possible.

2. Do the final cleaning with Calendula or Hypercal lotion mixed 1 to 20 parts water.

3. Cover and protect the wound if you think it is necessary.

4. When wound is dry and healing (if weeping use Hypercal lotion) you can use Calendula cream with maybe Comfrey cream as well for scar prevention or if the wound is healing slowly. You can also medicate a little bit of Calendula cream with Hypericum to make a Hypercal cream for a healing wound giving off nervy pain.

Homoeopathic Treatment

Hypercal - Which is a half and half mixture of Hypericum and calendula tinctures. you can use this to make lotions when you want the effects of both Calendula and Hypericum. A example on a human would be an infected crushed finger.

Creams - Calendula and Hypericum creams can be used when the healing begins and are applied for the same reasons as the lotions.

Arnica 6 to 30C - For shock, bruised sore pain of the wound, doesn't like effected area being touched.

Ledum 6 to 30C - Used for puncture wounds, prevents tetanus.

Puncture Wounds

Splinters and accidents from stepping on pins, rusty

nails, barbed wire or from tools can be dealt with very effectively with natural remedies.

Herbal Treatment

Hypercal Lotion - Externally use a lotion of Hypercal making sure plenty gets inside the wound so as to prevent tetanus. Other than this treat as a wound.

Homoeopathic Treatment

Arnica 6 to 30C - Can help bring splinters to the surface and deal with any shock.

Hypericum 6 to 30C - Intense pain shoots up from injured parts especially from those in nerve rich areas, if given immediately it can prevent tetanus from developing especially in puncture wounds of the hoofs but it is always best to get a booster shot.

Ledum 6 to 30C - This remedy also prevents tetanus and can be used for the same injuries as Hypericum but with Ledum the part feels cold and is relieved by cold, there is puffiness and a pale mottled appearance.

Herbal Overview Of The Skin

Conditions such as wounds, burns, bites, ticks etc. are all dealt with in First Aid For Animals which gives detailed treatment for these conditions. For problems such as Ringworm look to the Anti-Fungal and Anti Biotic herbs, also consider lotions such as Calendula with Garlic and Tea Tree oil in a spray bottle so as to soak the area and for easy application. For the long drawn out chronic diseases of the skin use the Alteratives especially the ones with a strong affinity to the skin such as Sarsaparilla, Burdock, Cleavers and Nettles. The blood cleansers need time to do their work so always consider using them for 3 months as this is the life cycle of the red blood cells so you would of cleaned most of the blood after using them for this time. For tumors think of Burdock.

Herbal Actions For The Skin

Alterative - Herbs that gradually restore proper function to the body, they increase health and vitality. They were once known as the blood cleansers.

Herbs - Black Cohosh, Blue Flag, Burdock, Cleavers, Chaparral, Echinacea, Fumitory, Garlic, Nettles, Pau D'Arco ,Sarsaparilla, Sweet Violets, Yellow Dock.

Anti-biotic - Echinacea, Garlic, Myrrh, Pau D' Arco, Tea Tree Oil

Anti-fungal - Marigold, Cats Claw, Pau D' Arco, Myrrh, Sweet Violets.

Anti-inflammatory - Helps the body to combat inflammations. Herbs mentioned under demulcents, emollients and vulnerary's will often act in this way especially when they are applied externally.

Herbs - Arnica, Blue Flag, Cats Claw, Chaparral ,Chickweed, Cleavers, Cranesbill, Chamomile, Eyebright, Ginger, Golden Rod, Guaiacum, Liquorice, Marshmallow, Marigold, Pau D' Arco, St Johns Wort, Sweet Violets, Witch Hazel.

Astringent - Contracts tissue which in turn reduces discharges, these herbs contain tannins.

Herbs - Agrimony, Bear Berry, Cranesbill, Chaparral, Chickweed, Comfrey, Eyebright, Golden Rod, Hops, Horsetail, Ladys Mantle, Marigold, Marshmallow, Meadowsweet, Myrrh, Nettles, Raspberry, Sage, Rosemary, Slippery Elm, Shepherds Purse, St Johns Wort, Slippery Elm, Thyme, Witch Hazel, Yarrow.

Emollient - Soothing to the skin. Acts externally the way demulcents do internally.

Herbs - Chickweed, Coltsfoot, Comfrey, Fenugreek, Liquorice, Marshmallow, Mullein, Plantain, Slippery Elm.

Parasiticide - Kills parasites and insects.

Herbs - Aniseed, Rosemary,

Vulnerary - Applied externally and aid the body in the healing of wounds and cuts

Herbs - Arnica, Burdock, Chickweed, Comfrey, Cranesbill, Elder, Fenugreek, Garlic, Horsetail, Hyssop, Marigolds, Marshmallow, Mullein, Myrrh, Plantain, Shepherds Purse, Slippery Elm, St Johns Wort, Thyme, Witch Hazel, Yarrow.

Circulatory And Blood Disorders

Heart Disease And Failure.

As the horse gets older the heart valves may get weaker or become blocked, or the heart may just get tired, other causes can be a bacterial or viral infection that damages the heart muscle or the sack surrounding the heart.

Signs of heart disease can include

1. A tendency to tire easily.
2. Breathlessness and heavy breathing.
3. A pale or bluish tinge to the gums.
4. Coughing especially early in the morning, wheezing, gasping and respiratory distress.
5. Exercise intolerance, tires easily, spends most of the day sleeping,
6. Restlessness, edgy, nervous, can't seem to get comfortable.

Herbal Treatment - Really depends on the cause.

If the cause is a bacterial or viral infection then the herbs to look at would be Echinacea, Myrrh and Garlic. If the cause is from old age then the herb would be Hawthorn.

Homoeopathic Treatment

Adonis 4X - This is one of the best remedies for valvular disease. Urine output is decreased and the urine contains albumen casts, the heart action is exaggerated, give one dose 3 times daily for 21 days.

Convallaria 4X - The pulse is full and intermittent, and the animal is disinclined to move, give 1 dose 3 times daily for 21 days.

Lillium Tig 6C - The pulse is small and rapid but weak when this remedy is indicated, even slight movement exacerbates the condition, sometimes acts better in the female, dose 3 times daily for 30 days.

Stropanthis 6X - Weakness of the heart muscle is accompanied by a quick pulse though sometimes irregular especially in pericarditis and scanty albuminous urine. The animal may show signs of pain on movement. Dose 3 times daily for 3 days.

Spongia 6C - Valvular incompetence with breathlessness and anxious expression, peripheral veins are prominent and there is usually a dry hard cough. Dose 3 times daily for 5 days.

Shock

Shock can result from injury (especially from loss of blood) or surgical interference and can lead to peripheral circulatory failure. Horses in shock are usually subdued, have pale membranes in their mouths and a fast weak pulse or heart rate of more than 70 beats per minute.

Signs and Symptoms

The skin becomes cold and the temperature falls to below normal, there is a fall in blood pressure and a weak pulse rate together with shallow respirations. Severe shock can lead to coma.

Herbal Treatment

Consider using Rescue Remedy from The Bach Flower Remedies.

Homoeopathic Treatment

Arnica 30C - This remedy should be given in all cases. Two doses usually suffice given 2 hours apart.

Bellis Perennis 200C - This is a useful remedy to combat shock after surgical intervention. Dose every 3 hours for 3 doses.

Carbo Veg 6C - Indicated in cases of collapse and threatened coma. Body surface is cold. Dose every 2 hours for 4 doses.

Veratum 200C - Useful in surgical shock and indicated when collapse is associated with cold perspiration. Dose every hour for 4 doses.

Haemorrhage

This may take several forms such as epistaxis, hemoptysis, wounds, birthing etc. and each case must be considered on its own symptoms.

Herbal Treatment

Calendula tincture diluted 1 to 10 can be used to stop bleeding in wounds and in heavy bleeding use the tincture and apply pressure to the wound.. Herbally you can use any astringents as these cause the blood vessels to spasm and contract which in turn stops the bleeding but make sure you choose a herb that is suited to the body system you are working on eg Ladys Mantle for the Reproductive System.

Homoeopathic Treatment

Ipecacuanha 30C - Useful when the blood is bright red and profuse. Dose every hour for 4 doses.

Phosphorus 200C - Indicated where there are

extravasations of blood in the skin and mucous membranes. Purpura like ecchymosis occur. Capillary bleeding is common. Dose 3 times daily for 3 days.

Ferrum Phos 6C - Indicated in febrile states and urinary tract involvement, blood is bright red. Dose every 2 hours for 4 doses.

China Off 30C - A useful remedy when there is extreme weakness and when slow leakage of blood is suspected. Dose every 2 hours for four doses.

Hamamelis 6C - Indicated in venous congestion with passive oozing hemorrhages. Dose 3 times daily for 2 days.

Edema

This is a term given to any abnormal amount of fluid in tissue spaces. It can arise from various causes.

Signs and Symptoms

Fluid swellings occur anywhere on the body surface and show pitting on pressure. The swellings may arise from some inflammatory condition or be dependent on poor peripheral circulation resulting from weak heart operation. Edema can also occur in body cavities such as the pleural and pericardial sacks.

Herbal Treatment

Here you have to know the cause to be able to choose the right herbs. If the cause is from a weak heart then Hawthorn is the herb. If you think the problem is urinary or a kidney problem then Dandelion Leaf is the herb as this is the best diuretic because it gives back more potassium then what your normal diuretic takes out, another good herb here is parsley.

Homoeopathic Treatment

Apis 6C - This is the main remedy for edematous states whether active from inflammation or passive as in chronic affections of the pleura and weak heart action. Dose 3 times daily for 3 days.

Ant Tart 6C - Indicated when edema affects the lung tissue, associated with great increase in mucous. Dose every 2 hours for 4 doses.

Digitalis 6C - Indicated if weak heart action is present. Dose 3 times daily for 5 days.

Anemia

This is the technical term for a deficiency of red blood cells or hemoglobin. The causes can be many some examples are blood loss from injury or maybe a heavy worm burden and sometimes it is caused by a blood disorder where tests have to be taken to see what's going on. In the diet iron, B12 and Folic Acid play an essential role in the makeup of the blood cells. Folic acid is found in plenty in fresh grass but disappears as a grass is made into hay so horses that spend a lot of time in the stables may be deficient here (feed alfalfa).

Signs and Symptoms - Anemia is characterized by pallor of the mucous membranes and a weak thready pulse. Jaundice and hemoglobinuria may occur. Weakness and lethargy are common. Appetite is depressed and the hair becomes dull and lifeless but it is not until the anemia becomes severe that the mucous membranes become pale.

Homoeopathic Treatment

China Off 30C - A useful remedy when there is extreme weakness and when slow leakage of blood is suspected. Dose every 2 hours for four doses.

Arsenic Alb 200C - This is a good remedy for long standing cases or pernicious anemia states, the animal is exhausted and restless, thirst is prominent for small quantities. Dose 3 times daily for 3 days.

Nat Mur 1M - Indicated in long standing cases depending on deficient salt metabolism, dose night and morning for 5 days.

Silicea 1M - When there is a increase in the number of white cells leading to interference in
hemoglobin function this is a very useful remedy. Dose twice weekly for 4 weeks.

Calc Phos 30C - This is a very useful remedy for the younger animal in the growing stage as it exerts a profound influence on the development of bone and muscle. More suitable for lean animals.

Purpura Haemorrhagica

This is a non-contagious disease that frequently follows other infectious diseases such as Strangles and other Streptococcal infections. This disease occurs 1 to 3 weeks after the horse appears to have recovered from the original infection. The cause is a allergic reaction to the break down products of bacteria circulating in the blood which in turn causes a bad reaction to the lining of blood vessels allowing blood to escape into the tissues.

Signs and Symptoms - Edema is the main symptom anywhere in the body especially in the legs. Blood stained fluid may ooze through the skin and there may be a stiffness or reluctance to move. Small hemorrhages may appear on the lips and the gums. There may be respiratory distress and swallowing difficulties due to fluid accumulation in the lungs and edema of the larynx. Other symptoms can be colic, blood stained diarrhea and anemia.

Herbal Treatment

This condition is a good example of why Echinacea should be used in acute diseases, not because of it immune boosting actions but in this case because of its action in cleaning up the blood along with its antibacterial action. Another herb to think of here is Burdock which is a alterative but also has a affinity to the spleen which is the bodies main blood cleansing organ. After a serious illness consider giving Fenugreek which is a good tonic (like a multivitamin if you see what's in it) but also has a gentle action on the lymphatic system stimulating the removal of rubbish. Another action to consider here is that of Antioxidants with a good example being Grapeseed which has affinity to blood vessels and may tone down the bad reaction of the blood vessels leading to the cause of the problem.

Homoeopathic Treatment

Apis 6C - This remedy is the specific for edematous

swellings and should be given as soon as they appear. Dose every two hours for 4 doses.

Phosphorus 200C - This is used for diseases and conditions where there is much bleeding, especially from mucous membranes. The remedy is more indicated when there are liver problems. This remedy is the specific for this disease. Dose three times daily for 3 days.

Kali Bich 30C - This may prevent further development of the edematous swellings. This remedy is also useful in controlling the oozing of serum from the swellings. Dose 3 times daily for 3 days.

Crotalus Horridus 200C - This is another specific for this condition with oozing of dark blood, again it is useful when there are liver problems. Dose four times daily for 2 days.

Lachesis 30C - Indicated when generalized petechial hemorrhages are accompanied by throat swelling and bleeding through the nose. Dose three times daily for 3 days.

Hamamelis 6C - Generalized venous congestion with enlarged throat veins. Purpura and petechiae are accompanied with pain. Dose three times daily for 3 days.

Sulphuric Acid 30C - Useful if the condition has arisen from strangles. Petechiae are associated with skin irritation. Dose once daily for 3 days.

Good Herbs To Use For Horses

Below are some good herbs for using on horses. Find a good herbal to use that not only gives you information about the herb but also tells you all the Actions the herb is capable of e.g. Astringent, Expectorant etc. It is very important to learn the actions of herbs so in times of need you can double or triple an Action required by using herbs in combination. Try not to use more than five herbs in any formula and always know exactly what each herb is being used for.

Aniseed - A good respiratory and digestive herb.

Astragalus - Immune booster for the more chronic diseases with fatigue.

Bladderwrack - (Kelp) - Helps the thyroid and supplies lots of minerals

Burdock - A cleansing alterative, good for skin conditions

Celery Seed - Rheumatoid Arthritis with mental depression, make a good supplement.

Chamomile - Gastro intestinal disturbance associated with nervous irritability. Colic.

Chaste Tree - A good hormone balancer especially for preparing for pregnancy.

Chickweed - Astringent, soothing to skin conditions. Use externally.

Cleavers - Lymphatic cleanser, has a high silica content.

Comfrey - Soothing demulcent to gastric ulcers, stimulates bone repair, full of minerals.

Dandelion - Toxic liver and digestive conditions. Blood cleanser.

Devils Claw - Inflamed joints and connective tissue. Anti-inflammatory and pain killing.

Dong Quai - Muscle damage and female reproductive disorders.

Echinacea - Any septic or infection condition or for a lowered immune system.

Elder - A good herb for the respiratory system.

Eyebright - Eye conditions and irritated mucous membranes, astringent, eye baths, allergies etc.

Fennel - Flatulence in foals and mares, the dieter herb (suppresses appetite), Colic.

Fenugreek - Debility and convalescence where digestion and nutrition poor, lymphatic cleanser.

Garlic - Give in any infection, don't use with sulphur drugs.

Ginger - Flatulent intestinal colic and any cold condition, arthritis.

Ginkgo Biloba - Any problem that can be traced to poor circulation.

Ginseng and Siberian - For a depressed immune system. Good for disease recovery.

Hawthorn Berry - A heart and circulation tonic.

Hops - A good nervine and digestive herb.

Lemon Balm - Tense behavior with digestive

problems, colic.

Licorice - Gastric upsets and heaves.

Marshmallow - Use the root for gastric ulcers. Leaf for respiratory catarrh. Both are demulcent.

Meadowsweet - Inflamed gastric mucosa and body aches and pains.

Motherwort - Anxious or nervous mares unable to cycle or badly behaved in season.

Mullein - Irritation to the airways and for painful dry coughs.

Nettle - Irritated skin conditions and eczema associated with nervous conditions.

Parsley - Flatulent dyspepsia with intestinal colic and helps with the urinary system.

Passion Flower - A Nervine and antispasmodic, useful for the horse that never relaxes.

Pau D`Arco - Any systemic disorder or general illness, strengthens the immune system.

Peppermint - Digestive problems, flatulence, pain, colic, colds, fevers.

Raspberry - Strengthens the uterus , astringent, diarrhea.

Rosehips - Dietary supplement as a natural source of vitamin C and small amounts of A and B.

Sage - Infections wounds of the mouth, respiratory infections especially of the throat.

Slippery Elm - Soothing demulcent that lines the digestive tract, diarrhea, nutrition.

St Marys Thistle - Any condition that requires liver support, antioxidant.

Valerian - Nervine relaxant, herbal tranquillizer.

White Willow - Rheumatoid arthritis and other systemic connective tissue disorders.

Wild Yam - Bilious colic and the acute phase of Rheumatism.

Wood Betony - Any complaint of the head region especially pain.

Yellow Dock - Skin diseases especially psoriasis with constipation.

Herbs To Avoid Using On Horses

Buckwheat (Fagopyrum Esculentum) All parts of the plant are toxic to horses and may cause blistering or peeling of the skin. It has caused photosensitivity in some animals.

Clovers can also be toxic to horses.

White Clover (Trifolium Repens) can cause laminitis so if your horse begins to show swelling or inflammation around the hooves check for this clover in the paddock.

Aliske Clover (Trifolium Hybridum) contains toxic nitrates and can cause blindness, depression and severe nephrosis as well as affecting your horses gait and triggering photosensitivity.

Red Clover (Trifolium Pratense) Can be feed in moderation and cause no harm but if ingested over a long period of time it may cause slobbering and digestive problems. It can sometimes induce abortion in mares.

Horsetail (Equisetum Arvense) Can cause a thiamine deficiency in horses. If mixed unknowingly in the hay in 2 weeks of feeding it may produce symptoms of weakness, staggering, muscle problems and diarrhea.

Melilot (Melilotus Alba) is closely related to clover and may cause anemia and hemorrhage in horses.

Onions wild and cultivated - Should be avoided by horses as they can cause weight loss and loss of appetite along with maybe discolored urine, muscle weakness, rapid breathing and a rapid heart rate.

St Johns Wort (Hypericum) - This herb contains Hypercin which once ingested spreads around the body via the circulatory system. Horses can have a severe reaction to this with symptoms of photosensitivity and peeling skin conditions that are extremely uncomfortable and slow to heal. The horse often rubs the area constantly until the skin is raw. If you accidentally feed your horse this herb or he grazes on it there may be symptoms of loss of appetite, mild fever and diarrhea and the gait may become irregular. In extreme cases a horse can suffer blindness or go into a coma. Small doses can be used reasonably safely in herbal formulas.

Herbal Supplement

Important Please Read

This Herbal Supplement is composed of the list Good Herbs For Horses. We are going to concentrate on these Herbs as they are fairly safe as are the doses mentioned. No doses were given for tinctures as the supplier should give the dose. Doses will vary along with the herb as some herbs are a lot stronger than others, a general rule to work by is to crush the herb and smell, the stronger the smell (the stronger the herb) the more essential oils the herb would have thus lessening the dose especially in a Extract or Tincture for they are made of alcohol solely for the reason of extracting those oils.

At the end of every section in the horse book for example The Digestive System there is an Overview of that section listing what are the common herbal actions needed for that system. The reason that is there is to teach you to think in the Actions you require for the treatment of your patient which gives you a more holistic view of the patient and what's happening. This makes you really start to think about what you are doing instead of thinking I will use the herb I used last time. Every case and every being is individual, think of what you are doing and why. Now for the hardest part, be patient, healing takes time. In the Actions explanation for example Demulcent, you will be told the meaning then given a list of herbs that are commonly known to be strong in that action, some will be different than what is listed in this herbal so you will have to do your own research but they should be generally safe for animal use as most of them come out of my Animal Herbal. Nearly all of the herbs mentioned have been historically used for animals and this is my part in making sure they are not forgotten again. I prefer using liquid to medicate in tinctures, extracts or infusion form even though there can be some controversy over the alcohol, the reason for this is that liquid spreads through the intestines a greater distance then the dry form which insures maximum absorption. In the herbal where no doses are mentioned these are the ones that are usually best in extract or tincture form and the manufacturers should give you the dose to match the strength that they have made it in.

Introduction To Herbal Medicine

Herbal Medicine has been in use and developed continuously since the beginning of time. It mainly evolved from observations from what plants did and the affects they had on people along with their animals. There is also what they call the Doctrine of Signatures which works like this, that flower really looks like a eye, maybe it helps sore eyes? I'll give it a try as my eyes are so sore and red. You know my eye really feels a lot better now, I think I will call that plant Eye Bright (Euphrasia) and tell my friends all about it especially my Dad who gets sore eyes to. In this way hundreds of plants were identified that have a medical action and no doubt there were also a lot of casualties.

The next great leap in herbal medicine was the Roman Empire of 2000 years ago. The Great Armies of Rome all had their own Medical Corps with Doctors, Battle Surgeons and Orderlies. It was these men who already had the knowledge of the Greeks that started to put together the best medical manuals in the world while at the same time started developing and using medical instruments and tools some of which are still used today. As the Romans conquered the known world more medicines and knowledge were found and assimilated.

The next great leap was modern Chemistry which allowed us to see exactly what herbs were made up of and what parts of the herb causes its medical action. Drug companies have made billions of Dollars from this information as they find the main active ingredient and then make a synthetic version of it, one good example that we all know of is Valium which is the synthetic version of the active ingredient from the herb Valerian. Leaving aside the Drug Companies let's see how Chemistry changed the way that modern herbalists think.

Modern science allows us to now know what Actions our herbs perform on the body so we shall carry on using Valerian as a example and see what Medical Actions Valerian has on the body.

The Actions of Valerian are Sedative, Hypnotic (sleep inducing), Anti Spasmodic (stops twitches, cramps etc.), Hypotensive (lowers Blood Pressure) and Carminative (calms and relaxes the tummy). Herbalists call Valerian the Herbal Tranquillizer and if you look at the above you can see why for if you can't sleep and your blood pressures up along with a gurgling tummy and a eye constantly twitching you definitely need to be calmed down.

The modern herbalist is trained to think in actions. There are many reasons for this but the main ones are to stop them from just using a handful of their favorite herbs and to train the mind to work in the method of thinking in actions that are needed. If we start thinking in the actions that are needed for a patient it makes us consider the problem in far more depth than just using our favorite herb and it forces our thinking to be far more holistic by taking in consideration the whole of the patient not just the part or the system we wish to treat.

Let's take a look at thinking in actions. The animal has a cough, but when it coughs it cant stop and the cough sounds a bit like whooping cough. The animal also sounds a little hoarse and the temperature is also elevated. The actions that come into mind for this are expectorant for the cough, anti spasmodics for the whooping quality of the cough and demulcents to sooth the sore throat. These are the obvious actions and we can add many more if we wish such as immune boosters for acute diseases, diaphoretics to reduce the temperature and prevent a fever and the list goes on. Next we look at how Herbal Actions are used in making Herbal Formulas.

Another point to make before we go to the formula making is that Professional Herbalists use Herbs in the form of Tinctures (water and alcohol solutions) as this allows them to mix formulas in any proportions that they like and also allows long term storage without spoiling.

Making Herbal Formulas

You should never have more the 5 Herbs in a herbal formula otherwise you start to lose track of what you are doing and how the formula is changing the symptoms. Always try to keep things simple. One of the herbs in the formula is used to force the formula into the body, to keep it simple we will only use three; they are Licorice, Ginger and Cayenne.

As an example let's use a animal with a cough. After further study of the case we decide that this is an Acute Disease for it came on quick and is fast acting not slow like a Chronic Disease. Listening to the animals cough we decide that it is a dry cough and upon looking at the animal's nose we can't see any mucus. Let's list the actions to consider.

Expectorants - Licorice, Aniseed, Fennel, Garlic and Mullein

Antispasmodics - Aniseed and Fennel

Demulcents - Licorice and Coltsfoot

Immune Boosters - Echinacea

Anti-Bacterial and Virals - Garlic and Echinacea

Out of the above I would choose Licorice, Echinacea,

Garlic, Aniseed and Fennel. I would make the formula in this strength.

Formula
Licorice - 20%
Garlic - 15%
Echinacea - 15%
Aniseed - 30%
Fennel - 20%

Look these herbs up in the herbal and consider why I used them, there are three obvious ones for Licorice alone with the first being to force the assimilation of the formula into the body, second is its expectorant action and third is its demulcent action in case the throat is sore and raw Next time you see a little kid eating heaps of licorice get them to open their mouth and look at their tongue which will be going black from the Licorice along with the throat etc. and know that you are looking at the demulcent action of Licorice working by coating and soothing.

The most important reason that you use the Actions Method for Herbal Prescribing is so that you can concentrate the Actions which are most needed for example, if it's a Bacterial infection concentrate on the Anti Bacterials, if it's a Viral infection concentrate on the Anti Virals, hopefully you are now beginning to see the importance of working in actions for if you don't concentrate a large part of the battle on the causes you may have lost the battle from the start.

Read through all the Actions listed in Herbal Actions at the end of each body system in the book and then do a study in depth of at least five Actions of your choice making the first two the Anti Bacterials and Anti Virals. Start trying to train your mind into thinking in Actions.

How To Make Herbal Tinctures

Tinctures are made by steeping the Herb plant material in a mixture of alcohol and water. Alcohol is usually always used at strength of 45%. The alcohol in this mixture will extract all the essential oils from the herb while the water will extract all that is water soluble, so between the both we are getting most of the medicinal properties out of the herb.

The proportions of herb to liquid are usually 1 part herb to 5 parts liquid. So find a suitable container (I use a big one liter preserving jar with a good sealing lid) and put into it 100grams of your chosen herb and to that add 500mls of our 45% solution of alcohol. Seal the lid and shake well for about a minute. Leave the jar on the window sill so the sun can shine on the jar for two weeks. The jar must be shaken for at least a minute every day.

After 2 weeks open and filter the contents of the jar. I use a large pouring jug into which I place a funnel and then place a coffee filter in the funnel and pour the jar contents through the funnel being careful not to let too much herb spill into the filter and block it up. When you get to the bottom of the jar you can crush the herb in your fist so as to extract the last of the liquid.

After this is completed you then get your chosen storage bottle, put a funnel into its neck followed by a coffee filter and then filter the jug into the bottle. Remember the solution should always be double filtered

Next we label the bottle, put the date, name and proportions e.g. 1 to 5 also state the recommended dose. Store in a cool and dark place. Most Professional Homoeopaths and Herbalists have access to pure alcohol so for them it is fairly easy to make tinctures while for the lay person they will probably have a hard time. An alternative is to use Vodka as strong as you can find it or find a way to twist the authorities arm into giving alcohol at 45% Don't even try to get pure alcohol as it is dangerous and can turn people blind and they won't give it to you.

How To Make Infusions

Infusions are a bit like making a cup of tea except we don't use milk. Infusions are used for the soft parts of the herb such as the flowers, leaves and fine twigs. The proportions for infusions are 1 to 20 e.g. 1 part herb to 20 parts water. Infusions are used for the more water soluble herbs.

Infusions can be made from a single herb or from a combination of herbs and may be drunk hot or cold. The water should be just off the boil before being poured on the herb and if you are making a infusion of a herb strong in essential oils such as Peppermint always cover the top of the cup to stop the essential oils from escaping in steam while the infusion is brewing. Allow up to 10 minutes to brew. It is best to make herbal teas fresh each day. You can experiment on yourself by getting Chamomile and Peppermint tea bags from the supermarket. Use honey as a sweetener.

How To Make Decoctions

Decoctions are used for the more hard woody substances of the herb such as barks, berries or roots. The process of decoction is far more vigorous then infusion as it involves heating the plant material in cold water, bringing it to the boil and simmering for 20 to 40 minutes. The finished ratio for decoctions is again 1 part herb to 20 parts water; remember to add more water at the beginning so you wind up with the 1 to 20 after steam loss. This form of preparation is no good for the herbs that are high in essential oils as these will all be lost in the steam.

How To Make Poultices

Poultices are used to sooth, irritate or draw impurities from the skin so choose your required plants by the actions you need. A Poultice is used to apply a remedy to the skin with moist heat and slight pressure. To prepare a poultice bruise or crush the fresh medicinal parts of the herb you are using into a pulpy mass and add a little hot water if needed. If using dried herb moisten the material by mixing with a hot soft adhesive substance such as moist flower and cornmeal or as they did in the past a mixture of bread and milk. This can be done to the fresh herb if you want as well. For ease of application to the skin it is best to spread the mixture on cheese cloth and fold to the appropriate size or shape required. The cloth also helps by retaining the moisture and even allows you to tie it gently the affected area. Moisten the cloth with hot water periodically when and if needed. Hot water bottles can also be used to keep the poultice warm. Always keep some cloth between the skin when using irritant plants such as mustard and always wash the skin thoroughly after use.

Dosage For Forms Of Herbal Medicines

Herbs can be given to animals in several different forms depending on what best suites the herb, the ailment, and the condition of the animal and of what is available at the time and then most importantly the expense. Most of the doses given are based on a full sized horse weighing about 600kg so adjust the dose accordingly to the size for example a Clydesdale draft horse would need a bit more while a Shetland pony may need under half the dose.

Herbal Extract - Are alcohol based and about the strongest herbal preparation you can get as they nearly extract everything from the herb. Generally the strength is every ml should be equivalent to one gram of the herb. Used and dosed the same as tinctures but the dose will always be less than what is used in a tincture. From this try to work out if the extra price is worth it. Supplier should give dosage.

Tincture - Is a weaker then Herbal Extracts but also made from alcohol. Dilute the appropriate number of drops in water for treatment. Supplier should give dosage.

Infusion - A infusion is like making a cup of tea out of the flowers and leaves and other soft parts of the herb. Add boiling water and cover so as all the essential oils don't escape in the steam and leave for 20 minutes. Afterwards strain and add 1 to 2 cupful's to the horses feed. A infusion or decoction is one of the easiest ways of dosing a horse.

Decoction - Usually made from the root, bark or seed and is simmered for a while to extract the medicinal properties. Usually dosed the same as infusions.

Powdered - These are usually made from roots and bark and given in doses from a teaspoon to tablespoon. These can also be infused and turned into a tea.

Fresh Herb - This is the easiest way to medicate a horse just add a large handful of the leaves to the feed. Always check for woody parts and sharp stalks. For dangerous or strong herbs chop finely and mix thoroughly into moistened feed so no one animal eats too much. Dose is usually a couple of handfuls.

Dried Herb - Most dried herb is usually cut, again run your hand through for wood or sharps. If you are growing the herb yourself cut up or grind and mix directly with the feed. Crushed herbs can also be mixed with water and formed into a pill for individual treatment or the whole stable can be dosed in a mix with feed. A cupful is usual the dose though give less for the stronger herbs. Dose up to 3 times a day depending on the severity of the condition and taking note of any of the warnings on the herb.

Note - Always be guided by the recommended dose of the individual herb instead of working in generals.

Notes

Herbal General Animal Doses
Common Herbal Dosages for Herbivores from Dr Hue Karreman

Form	*Goat*	*Cow*	*Horse*
Decoction	4oz	12oz	8oz
Extract Powder	1 tsp	2tbs	2tbs
Extract Tablet	3 to 5	10 to 15	10 to 15
Tincture	1 tsp	2 tbs	2 - 3 tbs

Herbivores require less per pound relative to the human or carnivore
Dosage. These doses are given two to three times daily.
Tbsp. = Tablespoon, roughly = to 15cc

Dr. Hubert Karreman is a 1995 graduate from the University Of Pennsylvania School Of Veterinary Medicine. He has been a dairy practitioner for 16 years in Lancaster, Pennsylvania. He is an internationally recognized expert in the non-antibiotic treatment of infectious disease.

Sheep - For sheep I would give a slightly smaller dose then that of the Goat as sheep are less hardy and have been severely genetically changed as I was trying to point out with my cover on the Sheep book.

Warning - Not all herbs in nature are of the same strength. For example if you gave the very strong herb Poke Root in tincture form at those doses the result would be a very sick animal, always remember herbs are not all the same. A safer way to go would be a comparison to the human dose to see if that is very low.

Notes

Calculating Correct Herbal Doses For Animals

Cats - 1/8 to 1/6 the dose for an adult human.

Dogs - Correspond to adult human dose according to weight.

Horse - 8 to 16 times the dose for an adult human.

Goats - 2 times the dose for an adult human.

Sheep - 1 1/2 times the dose for an adult human.

Cow - 12 to 24 times the dose for an adult human.

Swine - 1 to 3 times the dose for an adult human.

As mentioned in the warning above not all herbs are of the same strength so for this reason it is a good idea to always look at the human dose and if this dose seems to be lower than normal, if it is do your research into why. It might be a good idea to have a look at the herb Poke Root just to see what a strong herb looks like and can do.

Notes

Herbal

Aniseed

Actions - Expectorant, antispasmodic, carminative, parasiticide, aromatic.

Dogs like aniseed so much that it was once used as bait by dog thieves. As a carminative it is unsurpassed. A important remedy for all digestive ailments including colic.

Uses - Gripping, intestinal colic, wind, as a expectorant in bronchitis, tracheitis, irritable coughing, whooping cough

External - The oil by itself will help in the control of lice and scabies..

Dose - Average dose is one handful of seeds daily. (Must be for larger animals)

Astragalus

Actions - Immune-modulator, anti-viral, adaptogen, hypotensive, immune stimulant, adrenal tonic, diuretic, circulatory stimulant, vasodilator, blood tonic.

This herb should only be used in chronic diseases, as a preventative or in cases of fatigue especially in chronic diseases. Stimulates the natural production of interferon and intensifies the white cell destruction of germs.

A good tonic for strengthening the resistance to disease. Is very useful for animals in a state of chronic debility and fatigue by restoring the immune function. Use as a lung tonic to help expel toxins and pus in flu's, colds and sinusitis. Increases stamina and can accelerate wound healing, can help to replenish bone marrow. Strengthens the digestive system and aids adrenal gland function. This herb is used for cancer especially if the patient has had chemotherapy and helps aid them in their recovery.

Uses - Boosting immune system, disease preventative, fatigue, healing wounds. This is a good herb to use before and during a long distance or time consuming transportation.

Cautions - Should not be used in acute infections or fevers.

Burdock

Actions - Alterative, diuretic, bitter, antibacterial, anti-tumor.

It is used to treat conditions arising from an "overabundance" of toxins, such as boils, rashes and chronic skin problems. Helps to cleanse the body of waste products. Animals will not graze this herb with the exception of the ass, but the sliced and bruised roots are one of the finest blood cleansers known to herbalists. The bruised leaves applied externally are a remedy for ring worm and scabies. Soothing to the kidneys and a excellent diuretic. The juice is used internally for scabies and mites.

Uses - Remedy for all blood disorders, rheumatism, skin parasites , skin conditions resulting in dry scaly skin, psoriasis, eczema, dandruff, aids digestion and appetite, aids kidney function and helps with cystitis, speeds up the healing of wounds and ulcers. Use to reduce tumors.

Dose - In powdered form begin with one teaspoon full twice a day added to feed and can be increased to 2 teaspoons full twice a day if needed.

Celery Seed

Actions - Anti rheumatic, diuretic, carminative, sedative, alterative, hypotensive.

The main use for this herb is in the treatment of rheumatism, arthritis and gout. Celery seed can help soothe the nerves and relieve pain and also aids the body in the removal of uric acid. A good cleansing, mildly diuretic herb, useful in ridding the system of an accumulation of waste products. An improvement in circulation of fluids encourages a horse to drink and sweat more easily. Celery seed mixed with food aids in the digestion of protein. A very good digestive tonic if the horse is run down with little appetite.

Uses - Arthritis, hyperacidity, pain, hypertension, digestion, urinary tract infections

Dose - 1 tablespoon twice daily.

Chamomile

Actions - Carminative, sedative, anti-spasmodic, anti-inflammatory, analgesic and anti-septic.

It is a famed blood cleanser and pain reducer, reduces tumors (poultice), remedy for female ailments, inflamed gums, use for blood and skin disorders, aches and pains, external and internal inflammations, delayed menstruation, acid uterus and all female ailments, cleanser and toner of the digestive tract, it is well documented as having anti-inflammatory activity and is also beneficial in reducing allergic responses as it contains a number of anti-histamine chemicals. In addition, it is recognized as being ulcer-protective through its healing effect on the mucosa of the gastro-intestinal tract, expels worms and parasites, improves and helps appetite. Good for nervous and hyperactive horses as it calms them without making them tired.

Uses - Indigestion, colic, diarrhea, teething, anxiety, insomnia, nervous upsets, slowing down hyperactive horses, flatulence. Good all round tonic for the nervous system especially for nervous animals.

Dose -1 cup of infusion added to feed twice a day or a hand full of flowers replacing the infusion.

Chaparral

Actions - Alterative, astringent, diuretic, tonic, powerful antioxidant, anti-arthritic, anti-rheumatic, anti-cancer, anti-tumor, dissolves calculi, anti-biotic.

Uses - Used in kidney problems and stones and for rheumatism and arthritis. Aids in healing skin blemishes, acne, allergies, promotes hair growth, acts as a natural antibiotic, cataracts, has a action on cancer.

Chaste Tree

Actions - Emmenagogue, galactagogue, Tonic for the reproductive organs.

More of a hormone balancer by working directly on the pituitary gland though is more of a normalizing herb, usually increases the progesterone levels therefore increasing the chance of pregnancy. Supporting the progesterone level is extremely helpful in counteracting the irritability and unpredictability that can happen with mares in season making them more comfortable, cooperative and safer to handle. Though this herb is primarily used to balance hormonal irregularities in mares it can also be used to inhibit the sex hormones of stallions if their behavior is thought dangerous or seen to be causing them a loss in condition. Useful on its own or in combination with herbs specific for hormonal balance.

Used for endometriosis, fibroids, infertility and threatened miscarriages.

Chickweed

Actions - Healing, anti-inflammatory, astringent, emollient.

Rich in copper, highly tonic food for the digestive system and a remedy for all stomach ailments, allergies, colon problems, constipation, piles, rheumatism, skin problems, eczema, psoriasis, itching, irritation, cuts and wounds.

Uses - One of the main uses of this herb is for itching skin conditions whether from insect bites or eczema like conditions. Has wound healing and demulcent properties.

Dose - Usually given in infusions or used as a lotion or cream.

Cleavers

Actions - Alterative, diuretic, anti-inflammatory, astringent, tonic, anti-cancer.

A lymphatic tonic with alterative and diuretic actions which can be used in a wide range of problems where the lymphatic system is involved. The plant is very rich in minerals and silica, gives good strong texture to the hair of animals and strengthens the hoofs. Also used to ease swollen legs and joints, support the lymphatic and endocrine systems and encourage the elimination of toxins, is also helpful if your horse experiences muscle tightening during or after exercise. All animals eat it and poultry especially seek it hence its popular name of goose grass. Good for skin ailments.

Uses - Tonic, eczema, abscesses and tumors, cancerous growths, swollen glands, tonsillitis, psoriasis, cystitis.

Dose - 1 cup full daily or 2 tablespoons full of powder daily.

Comfrey

Actions - Demulcent, astringent, healing, expectorant.

Once widely cultivated as a fodder plant, sheep and cows eat it greedily, the impressive wound healing powers of comfrey are partially due to allantoin which stimulates cell proliferation and speeds the healing process inside and out. Has been used for thousands of years as a herb with abilities to mend broken bones. Has the same result on wounds, tendons, fractures, sprains, ulcers and cartilage.

Uses - Its old name is knit bone and that describes well what it does. Comfrey also guards against scar tissue from developing incorrectly, all internal hemorrhages including uterine, reunion of wound and fractures, internal ulcers, ruptures, pulmonary problems, bronchitis, irritable cough, ulcerative colitis, skin ulcers and varicose veins.

Dose - Half a cup of the cut herb up to 3 times daily.

Dandelion

Actions - Diuretic, cholagogue, anti-rheumatic, laxative, tonic

The leaves of the Dandelion plant are generally fed to horses during spring as the herb assists with cleansing the blood. They are high in iron and calcium as well as Vitamins A, B, and D and are traditionally used as a tonic to stimulate the bladder.

The herb is blood cleansing and tonic, it has an

important effect on the hepatic system and is a supreme jaundice curative herb, the leaves strengthen the enamel of the teeth and the white   juices of the freshly crushed stem dissolves warts, the plant is well grazed by goats, horses will take quantities of the leaves when cut and well mixed with bran. Dandelion Root is helpful for horses recovering from an illness or a reaction to vaccination. Being a tonic, this herb assists to clean the liver, kidneys and blood and is high in potassium and magnesium. Excellent for anemia because it is high in iron, calcium, copper and vitamins, useful in kidney and bladder problems, skin eruptions, sluggish blood flow, weak arteries, all liver complaints, jaundice, constipation, gallbladder problems and rheumatism.

Dose - 2 tablespoons of powder daily or make as infusion and pour over feed.

Devils Claw

Actions - Anti-inflammatory, pain killer, hepatic, anti-rheumatic, alterative.

Used for its analgesic and anti-inflammatory properties, it is useful for treating pain in a range of joint and muscular problems. The bitter action of Devils Claw stimulates and tones the digestive system. Good for reducing inflammation in arthritis, gout and rheumatism. Aids the body in the elimination of uric acid. This plant also aids liver and gallbladder complaints.

Dose - 1 tablespoon of powder twice a day or more

in severe conditions but only for a short time.

Caution - Use with demulcent herbs to save irritating the tummy, don't use on horses with ulcers.

Dong Quai

Actions - Emmenagogue, antispasmodic, analgesic, uterine tonic ,vasodilator, hormone balancer, alterative.

Known regulator for the female reproductive system. Some of its compounds stimulate the uterus while others relax the uterus. The compounds that stimulate the uterus are water soluble and are absorbed into the body from teas and capsules. The compounds that relax the uterus are soluble in alcohol and are provided by tinctures. This herb may stop cramping, and ease the pain of ovarian cysts. The Chinese use this herb for abnormal menstruation, suppressed flow, painful or difficult menstruation. This herb is also good for the treatment of psoriasis. Dong Quai also helps with asthma, bronchitis, emphysema and improves the function of the lungs. Builds and improves circulation as well as disperses congestion in the pelvic area.

Dose - 1 to 3 teaspoon full per day depending on severity of the condition.

Cautions - Avoid during pregnancy and in cases with diarrhea and dysentery.

Echinacea

Actions - Immune stimulant, anti-microbial, anti-inflammatory, alterative, healing.

Is an infection fighter active against strep bacteria (abscesses and boils), a blood cleanser, (blood poisons, snake bites, poisonous insects) and a glandular and lymphatic system cleanser. Use it particularly for respiration infections and for any disease above the waist. This is one of our main immune boosters for the acute diseases. Use as a prophylactic to protect horses from infections especially when traveling.

Uses - All infections, depressed immune function, inflammatory conditions, allergies, effective against both bacteria and viruses.

Dose - half to 1 tablespoon 3 times daily or half a cup dry leaf or shaved root up to 3 times daily depending on the severity of the condition. Infusions can be used to.

Warning - Do not use continually as you will burn out the immune system give a few weeks break after 3 weeks. Beware also in the use of allergies for you could be building up the immune system just to attack itself.

Elder

Actions - Diaphoretic, diuretic, anti-catarrhal, expectorant.

Most animals will graze on elder. Used for the

treatment of all gastric, hepatic, and pulmonary ailments, all fevers, skin disorders especially scabies and ring worm, externally as a insecticide.

Leaves - Externally emollient and vulnerary (bruises, sprains and wounds). Internally used as a purgative, expectorant, diuretic and Diaphoretic. Topically the lotion makes a anti-inflammatory wash, salve, eyewash and gargle for sore throats.

Flowers - Diaphoretic and Anti catarrhal. Use for colds and flu.

Berries - Diaphoretic and Anti catarrhal. The uses are similar to the flowers but the berries are used for rheumatism. The berries have been used as a nutrient rich tonic given after birth to help build the blood.

Dose - Really depends on which part of the plant you are using the leaves, flowers or berries.

Eye Bright

Actions - Anti-inflammatory, astringent, anti-catarrhal.

As the name says this is one of the main herbs in the treatment of eye problems. The aerial (above ground) parts of the plant are used. As its name suggests, it helps eye problems by relieving inflammation and tightening mucous membranes and is specifically used in treating conjunctivitis and blepharitis. Used for infections and allergic conditions affecting the eyes, middle ear, sinuses and nasal passages.

The plant is also nervine, tonic and astringent. Its use

is both internal and external strengthening greatly the eyes nerves when used so. The high potassium and sulphur content of the plant make it also of value in treatment of gastric ailments especially insufficiency of gastric juices. Acts as a internal medicine for the constitutional tendency to eye weakness.

Uses- Best known for its use in the eye where it is helpful in acute or chronic inflammations, stinging and weeping eyes, over sensitivity to light, conjunctivitis, allergies, sinusitis, ulcers and general eye weakness.

Dose - 1 teaspoon of powdered herb or half a cup of dried herb morning and night.

Fennel

Actions - Carminative, aromatic, anti-spasmodic, stimulant, galactagogue, expectorant.

The herb possesses highly antiseptic and tonic properties. The primary use of fennel is to relieve bloating, but it also settles stomach pain, stimulates the appetite and is diuretic and anti-inflammatory. Peasants drive their flocks to feed upon it owing to the abundance of milk that the herb produces and the sweet odor that it imparts upon the milk. (if the animal is not native they can over gorge and poison themselves).

Arabs use fennel poultices to resolve old and hard tumors.

Uses - Gastric ailments, relieves flatulence and colic, stimulates appetite, inflammation of the bowels, acute constipation (raw roots daily), fevers, cramps, worms, indigestion, all eye ailments, bronchitis, coughs, muscular and rheumatic pains use the oil. Externally used as an eye wash to treat eye infections.

Dose - One tablespoon of seeds given twice daily.

Fenugreek

Actions - Expectorant, demulcent, tonic, carminative, galactagogue, alterative, restorative.

Strongly aromatic herb and the seeds of the plant are used. It contains a volatile oil, flavonoids, mucilage, protein, Vitamins A, B & C, alkaloids, saponins and some minerals. The seeds can aid in recovery from illness and to encourage weight gain. This is a herb well worth getting to know not just because of its tonic properties but for its rubbish removing actions especially in mucous thick chronic diseases such as sinusitis. Always use cleansing herbs like this one slowly and at low doses especially when using for long periods of time. The plant possesses highly aromatic seeds having a powerful disinfectant, emollient and lubricant properties. The feeding value of these is about equal to linseed. It is one of the great fattening herbs. The perfect sister herb for garlic enhancing all its powers. Very tonic and eagerly sought by all animals. Rich in vitamins and nitrates, calcium and phosphorus. The whole plant is used.

Uses - Treatment for all gastric weaknesses and ailments, nerves and neuralgia, female ailments including failing milk supply, allergies, bronchitis, anemia, bruises, colitis, coughs, diabetes, fever, flu, hay fever, headache, migraines, lung problems, sinus congestion, ulcers, reduces inflammation, has a reputation for stimulating and developing breasts.

Externally - It can be used as a poultice for relief of abscess, boils, tumors and running sores.

Dose - One to two handfuls of plant feed a day, to obtain a quicker result use the seed - 2 tablespoons of seed daily. Use seed for the poultices.

Caution - Avoid during pregnancy as it can be a uterine stimulant.

Garlic

Actions - Immune stimulant, anti-bacterial, anti-viral, anti-fungal, anti-septic, anti-oxidant, diaphoretic, cholagogue, hypotensive, anti-spasmodic, vermifuge and many more.

The plant is rich in volatile oil and sulphur and because of its remarkable penetrating, disinfecting and mucous expelling powers garlic is a valuable basic remedy for the treatment of all ailments in which the cleansing of the blood stream and expulsion of mucous accumulations is required. Garlic can be used to prevent and treat respiratory infections. Anyone who has had garlic breath has experienced this herb's aromatic compounds being excreted through their lungs which is why garlic's active ingredients can be so effective for respiratory complaints. Garlic is extremely effective in dissolving and cleansing cholesterol from the blood stream, it stimulates the digestive tract, kills worms, parasites and harmful bacteria, normalizes blood pressure, reduces fever, gas and cramps.

Uses- All infections, coughs, colds, flu, bronchitis, all fevers, pulmonary conditions, gastric and skin complaints, rheumatism, all worms and also liver fluke, mange, ringworm, ticks and lice.

Acts on Bacteria, Viruses and Internal Parasites.

Dose - 1 clove every second day as maintenance. Two cloves a day in sickness but for only a couple of weeks.

Externally - You can use garlic for ring worm and ear ache, to disinfect wounds and sores, parasitical infections.

Ginger

Actions - Carminative, anti-inflammatory, vasodilator, circulatory stimulant, diaphoretic, anti-emetic.

The therapeutic benefits of ginger are largely due to its volatile oil and oleoresin content. Ginger is an excellent remedy for many digestive complaints, including nausea, colic, wind and indigestion. Its antiseptic properties also make it beneficial for gastro-intestinal infections. For the older, arthritic horse, ginger is a useful maintenance herb. It stimulates the circulatory system and helps blood flow and increases stamina. Aids in fighting colds, colitis, digestive disorders, wind, increases saliva.

Uses- Indigestion, nausea, feverish conditions especially when chills are present, travel sickness especially sea sickness, dyspepsia, colic, flatulence.

Dose - In powder form 1 tablespoon twice a day or 1 tablespoon of grated 3 times a day or an infusion over feed 3 times a day.

Caution - Don't use large doses on a empty stomach..

Ginkgo Biloba

Actions - Anti fungal, anti-bacterial, antioxidant, anti tussive, astringent, expectorant, anti-allergy and anti-inflammatory but mainly used for its Peripheral Vaso - Dilator effects.

Is native to Northern China and is considered the world's oldest tree species. This herb can be helpful for a horse resuming work after a spell, or for older horses that are sound for riding but are slowing down. Due to its effect on peripheral and cerebral (brain) circulation it can assist the blood supply to limbs, and general alertness. (think of mixing with Hawthorn). The leading symptoms pointing to Ginkgo are cold hands and feet. This herb opens up the femoral arteries and neck arteries increasing blood supply to those areas thus improving the function of everything in those areas by the increase in oxygen and blood sugar. For the old animal thinking and seeing may improve and walking may also become a bit easier. In asthma ginkgo helps reduce the inflammation response making the attacks less severe.

The herb is safe to use as a tonic. This is a good herb to take in a mixed antioxidant formula.

Dose - 1 cup full twice daily of the cut leaf.

Ginseng (Panax)

Actions - Anti depressive, restorative, tonic, adaptogen, stimulating adrenal agent, increases resistance and improves mental and physical performance.

This is the strong ginseng, think twice about giving it to a horse with a shy and sensitive nature it's more for the outgoing and competitive nature. This herb can help with depression especially when caused by debility and exhaustion. It can be used in general for exhaustion and weakness. Used to increase mental and physical performance, to improve concentration, vigilance and work efficiency, stamina, for combating internal or external stress factors of any kind - athletics, endurance activities, aging, surgery, disease, infections, cold, but especially degenerative conditions and problems of old age. This is a good herb for infertility.

Doses - 1 teaspoon full of powdered herb and see what happens.

Cautions - Avoid with high blood pressure, during acute infections. This herb can be over stimulating for some. Use month on month off.

Ginseng Siberian

Actions - Adaptogen, vaso dilator, increases stamina, circulatory stimulant.

This herb is very similar to the one above but is a milder version and can be used all the time as it does not build up in the system like Panax Ginseng. Always consider giving a break from herbs as it is not good to use any herb all the time except maybe Hawthorn for a failing heart.

Dose - 1 teaspoon full in the feed up to 3 times a day.

Hawthorn

Actions - Cardiac tonic, hypotensive, adaptogen.

Strengthens the muscles and nerves of the heart, aids in relieving emotional stress, regulates high and low blood pressure, helps combat arteriosclerosis and heart disease. With regard to horses, hawthorn's effects on peripheral circulation makes it valuable for treating conditions such as navicular and laminitis. Indeed, horses and ponies suffering from these ailments have been observed seeking out the new growth on hawthorn bushes. This more of a balancing herb, if the blood pressure is high or low the herb will balance it if the electrical activity is playing up with rapid or erratic heart beat it will try to balance it. Strengthens and helps to remove plaques from the blood vessels. This is a herb for taking in the long term.

Uses - As a tonic to the circulatory system and to

strengthen the heart.

Dose - 2 tablespoons of the powdered berry 3 times daily mix in the feed.

Hops

Actions - Sedative, hypnotic, antiseptic, astringent, nervine, bitter digestive tonic, antibacterial.

Famed for its tonic and nervine properties, pain reliever, sleep inducer, anti-septic, vermifuge, tension that leads to restlessness, headache, indigestion, mucous colitis. Good for when digestive problems are caused by worry or nerves. Good for nervous horses. One of the main remedies for IBS. Acts on the central nervous system and calms and eases anxiety. Hops contains estrogenic substances which could interfere with hormone therapy.

Uses - Treatment of all digestive ailments, general debility, failing appetite, wasting, fevers, eczema, worms, to quietens restless animals.

Externally - Eczema.

Kelp

Actions – Anti-hypothyroid, anti-rheumatic, nutritive,

Used mainly for under active thyroid (iodine) especially when it is thought to be the cause of overweight. Helps in the relief of rheumatism internally and externally. Added to feed for nutrition. Can be used to slim fat horses. Make sure that iodine isn't in any of the supplements you are already giving. It is good for coat and hoof conditions.

Dose - 2 tablespoons a day for overweight horses half the amount for normal.

Lemon Balm (Melissa)

Actions - Carminative, antispasmodic, anti-depressive, diaphoretic, hypotensive, emmenagogue, nervine, rejuvenating tonic, Anti-viral.

In the past this plant was used to attract bees by rubbing it all around a new hive and the smell made the bees want to stay. The name Melissa is Greek for honey bee. The Arabs say it gives intelligence to any animal that feeds upon it.

Relieves spasms in the digestive tract and is used in flatulent dyspepsia. Good for digestive problems brought on from worry, anxiety and stress. Has a tonic effect on the heart and circulatory system causing mild vasodilatation of the peripheral blood vessels which can help to lower blood pressure and also may calm the electrical activity of the heart. Has also been used in animals for retained afterbirth and as an anti-viral for infections such as herpes.

Dose - 1 cup full of dried herb twice daily.

Caution - Can sometimes lower thyroid function.

Licorice

Actions - Expectorant, demulcent, anti-inflammatory, adrenal agent, anti-spasmodic, mild laxative.

The root part is used , possessing unique pectoral and emollient properties, it is also nutritive and slightly laxative, It contains the building blocks of hormones, has a marked effect on the endocrine system, catarrh, gastric and peptic ulcers, abdominal colic. Its ability to soothe irritated mucous membranes and to break up phlegm and ease coughing sees licorice employed in respiratory conditions, coughing, bronchitis, and chest colds. Can be used for treating inflammatory and allergic conditions.. Licorice has effects on the adrenal glands which are protective, restorative, tonic and stimulatory. These properties can aid the horse which is recovering from steroid therapy or abuse.

Uses - Treatment of cough, inflamed throat, pneumonia, pleurisy, TB, all catarrhal conditions, gallstones, chronic constipation, mild worms in young animals, female infertility, pains of colic.

Dose - 1 teaspoon full of powder daily.

Caution - Do not use with high blood pressure. Long term use depletes potassium which raises the blood pressure. Don't use with steroids.

Marsh Mallow

Actions - Demulcent, anti-inflammatory, expectorant, astringent.

Its therapeutic effects are largely due to its significant mucilage and pectin content, aided by its anti-inflammatory properties. The foliage of the mallow is eaten by all animals, the roots are the main part used for internal medicine and also the leaves which are especially used for inflammation of the stomach and bowel and especially used for ulcers, it contains over half its weight in sweet tasting mucilage which has unique properties of lubricating, soothing and healing. A poultice can be used for all inflammatory conditions. Horses who have colic, or who are scouring, can benefit from the soothing and healing effects of marshmallow also see Slippery Elm. Consider using as a supplement for horses prone to colic and ulcers. Marshmallow can also be used to soothe inflamed and irritated mucous membranes of the respiratory and urinary systems. Dry coughs, sore throats, urinary tract inflammation and cystitis have all been relieved by the effects of marshmallow.

Uses - Treatment of sore throats, pulmonary catarrhs, pleurisy, cystitis, diarrhea, dysentery, ulcers, bowel inflammations and hemorrhages.

Externally - All skin eruptions, abrasions, swellings, inflammations, bruises, sore inflamed udders.

Dose - 1 to 2 hands full infused. Give 1 cup twice a day. 2 tablespoons of the powdered root 2 to 3 times daily.

Meadowsweet

Actions - Anti-inflammatory, anti-rheumatic, antacid, anti-emetic, stomachic, astringent.

A important fever and diarrhea herb, the gypsies use as a spring tonic for their animals, eaten plentifully by goats and sheep, acts to protect and soothe the mucous membranes of the digestive tract reducing excess acidity and easing nausea, heart burn, hyperacidity, gastritis, peptic ulcers. This herb is a good acid balancer and is good for correcting over acid systems. Meadowsweet is the forerunner of aspirin as this is the first herb it was synthesized from in 1835 but as this herb contains its own buffering agents it is gentle on the stomach. Used to help reduce inflammation and for pain relief in case of arthritic conditions. Useful alone or in combination with other herbs for effective pain management.

Uses - Fevers, arthritis, diarrhea and the above mentioned.

Dose - 1 cup full of dried flowers twice daily.

Caution - Avoid if sensitive to salicylates.

Motherwort

Actions - Sedative, emmenagogue, antispasmodic, cardiac tonic.

As its species name indicates, it has long been considered a nerve and heart remedy. It strengthens heart function, particularly where it is weak. Antispasmodic and sedative, the herb causes relaxation rather than drowsiness. Motherwort is considered a life giving plant, beneficial for all female disorders and a general heart tonic. Delayed or suppressed menses especially where anxiety or tension are involved, specific for over rapid heartbeat brought on by anxiety or tension, lowers high blood pressure and is used for the pains of birth and given for a few days after so as to prevent bleeding and infection.

Dose - 1 cup full of the leaf given daily.

Mullein

Actions - Expectorant, demulcent, mild diuretic, mild sedative, vulnerary.

The herb is famed for its powers in pulmonary ailments being much used in lung ailments of cattle, a bone flesh and cartilage builder, aids in healing respiratory ailments, asthma, bronchitis, sinus congestion, soothing to any inflammation and relieves pain, acts to relieve spasms and clears the lungs, tones mucous membranes of the respiratory system, inflammation of the trachea, painful coughs. The leaves of Mullein were traditionally fed to animals that cough especially horses.

Uses - Coughs, pneumonia, bronchitis, pleurisy, TB, asthma, diarrhea, internal bleeding of the lung and bowel.

Dose - 1 cup full of herb daily added to feed.

Nettles

Actions - Astringent, diuretic, galactagogue, tonic, nutritive.

Nettle is perhaps best known as a highly nutritious feed herb/fodder for animals, and has been used through the ages for this purpose. It is considered a spring tonic and detoxifier for human and animal alike. One of the richest sources of chlorophyll in the vegetable kingdom, rich in iron, lime, sodium, Vit C, chlorine and contains much protein. Preventative against many ailments, increases milk yield, fattener for poultry. Good astringent for stopping bleeding anywhere but especially in the urinary tract. Good for eczema in the young especially in the nervous young. Good for pregnant and nursing mothers. The seeds can be used as a thyroid tonic.

Uses - Treatment of wasting diseases, poor appetite, lung disorders, blood impurities, worms, fever, cold, hay fever, allergies, eczema, diarrhea, hemorrhage.

Externally - Paralysis, rheumatism, arthritis, loss of muscular power.

Dose - 1 cup full of herb 2 to 3 times daily.

Caution - Only buy the product prepared for herbal use.

Parsley

Actions - Diuretic, carminative, emmenagogue, expectorant.

Well-liked by sheep and goats, improves their milk yield and keeps them free from foot ills. It is a great enricher of the blood being very rich in iron and copper. Nutrient, digestive tract tonic, diuretic, high in potassium minerals and vitamins, bladder and kidney infections, incontinence, blood cleanser, immune builder, tonic for the blood vessels, aids in afterbirth pains, mainly used as a diuretic, carminative and emmenagogue. Is a good source of chlorophyll, parsley is useful for combating bad breath. Its diuretic properties are beneficial in: arthritic/rheumatic conditions associated with poor kidney function; urinary infections; kidney and bladder stones. Parsley also acts as a digestive tonic by easing spasms and minimizing flatulence.

Uses - Treatment of all disorders of the kidneys and bladder, gravel, stones, congestion, cystitis, jaundice, obesity, dropsy, worms, rheumatism, prostrate problems, sciatica, swellings of the joints, the root can be used for constipation and obstructions of the intestines.

Dose - 1 cup of dried herb twice daily.

Caution - Do not use in pregnancy.

Passion Flower Incarnata

Actions - Sedative, antispasmodic, anodyne, relaxant, epilepsy, shingles, asthma, hypotensive.

A good herb for insomnia and a very effective herb for nerve pains especially in conditions like shingles. This herbs focus is more on restlessness and irritability, hysteria and anxiety and is soothing to the mentally worried and overworked it acts on nervousness especially due to unrest, agitation, worry, exhaustion and cerebral excitement. Can be of benefit to horses that are generally nervous and apprehensive. Used in the treatment of convulsions, epilepsy, tremors, hypertension, nervous breakdowns, migraines and neuralgias.

Doses - 2 teaspoons of powdered herb daily or half a cup of herb daily.

Cautions - Large doses may cause nausea and vomiting. Do not use while pregnant.

Pau D'Arco

Actions - Alterative, anodyne, analgesic, antifungal, antibacterial, anti-inflammatory, antioxidant, antiviral, diuretic, immune stimulant.

This herb comes from Brazil and is used by the Indians there. It possesses properties that are antibiotic, tumor inhibiting, virus killing, anti-fungal and anti-malarial. Builds up the immune system. Its anti-inflammatory action applies especially in the stomach and intestines as well as for conditions such as cystitis, inflammation of the cervix, arthritis and prostatitis; it is a good herb for fighting fungal infections while building up the immune system. This herb is used for lung, colon and prostate cancer. It contains a chemical called lapachol that inhibits tumor cell growth by preventing them from metabolizing oxygen. Pau D'Arco also lowers blood sugar levels and acts as a mild laxative.

Dose - 1 to 2 teaspoons of powdered herb daily.

Peppermint

Actions - Carminative, diaphoretic, anti-spasmodic, anti-emetic, nervine, analgesic, anti-septic.

Best known for its ability to aid digestion and relieve

gastrointestinal distress. Peppermint owes most of its medicinal value to menthol, which is cooling, anesthetic, antiseptic and soothing to the stomach. For horses, peppermint's aroma is useful for tempting fussy eaters and/or helping to mask the smell of less pleasant herbs in their feed. It eases flatulence/bloating, increases the flow of bile from the liver and relaxes both gastrointestinal spasms and tight skeletal muscles.

Uses- Nausea, heartburn, indigestion, colic, flatulence, dyspepsia, vomiting, fevers, migraine headaches and irritable bowel syndrome (IBS) and for travel sickness think of adding Ginger for this.

Dose - 1 to 2 cups of dried herb daily.

Caution - May reduce milk flow if breast feeding.

Raspberry

Actions - Astringent, tonic, refrigerant, parturient.

Raspberry leaf has been used for mares with oestrus problems and the attendant behavioral disturbances. For mares that have had or may have difficulty conceiving it can be given for a period prior to mating. Generally, raspberry leaf is used to tone the uterine muscles, encourage an easy labor, and hemorrhaging during and after birth

Highly tonic and cleansing improving the condition of the organism during pregnancy ensuring speedy and strong expulsion of the fetus at birth, use as a drench in retained afterbirth, acclaimed as a tonic for male animals and as a cure for sterility, becomes especially potent for female use when blended with feverfew - 3 parts to 1 part of feverfew. As a astringent it can be used in diarrhea and leucorrhoea, it is valuable in easing mouth problems such as mouth ulcers, bleeding gums and inflammations

Uses - Prevention and treatment of all female ailments, retained afterbirth, digestive ailments including diarrhea, treatment of mouth and throat ailments as a gargle.

Dose - 1 cup full daily.

Rose Hips

Actions - Nutrient, mild laxative, mild diuretic, mild astringent.

The foliage is enjoyed by all animals. The flowers are tonic and astringent. The fruits are slightly aperient and rich in vitamin C. A good spring tonic and aid to general debility and exhaustion. Used to fight infection and curb stress. Rosehips are often fed to horses recuperating from injury as they help to restore the immune system and aid tissue repair and leaking capillaries with their bioflavonoids.

Dose - 1 cup full of infusion twice daily.

Sage

Actions - Carminative, antispasmodic, antiseptic, astringent.

Sage is well liked by animals and as with other aromatics makes the milk refreshing, tonic and increases the milk yield, it is a nervine, digestive and blood cleanser, a first rate remedy for all disorders of the throat, lungs and ears, inflamed and bleeding gums, inflamed tongue or general mouth inflammation, mouth ulcers, a good mouth wash.

Uses - Treatment of nerve debility, paralysis, all gastric ailments, constipation, obesity and female ailments, eczema, fevers, wound infections.

Dose - Infuse 1 teaspoon of powdered herb in 2 cups of water. Use in small doses. For sore mouths and throat ailments give mixed with honey.

Caution - Stimulates the muscles of the uterus so should be avoided during pregnancy.

Slippery Elm Bark Powder

Actions - Demulcent, emollient, nutrient, astringent. Slippery elm bark provides a nutritious gruel which also possesses remarkable medicinal properties acting as a poultice both internally and externally. A nutrient and food for very old or young or weak especially if mixed with honey, coats and heals all inflamed tissues internally and externally and is used for the stomach, intestines, ulcers, ulcerative colitis, enteritis, dysentery, constipation and internal bleeding of the digestive tract.

Uses - Treatment of all digestive complaints especially ulcers for which it is a specific, dysentery, all pectoral disorders including TB, lung and bronchial hemorrhage, wasting diseases, rickets, stunted growth. Calves with scour can be kept alive on this mixed with honey while the non-treated can die.

Externally - A poultice for all skin ailments especially old ailments and hard swellings.

Dose - Mix 2 tablespoons of powder with honey to form a paste and dose orally or blend with a cup of water.

St Mary's Thistle - Milk Thistle

Actions - Cholagogue, galactagogue, demulcent.

This herb is said to rejuvenate the liver, for problems like hepatitis it is used alone at first as it drains the liver probably by its action of stimulating the gallbladder to release bile. Much of the therapeutic benefit of the seeds is attributed to a group of potent antioxidant bioflavonoids, known together as silymarin, which are able to guard and stabilize cell membranes, preventing the invasion of toxins, as well as enhance the regeneration of liver cells already damaged by detoxification processes. for horses who have suffered liver damage from poisons, infections, high worm burdens, reactions to worming drugs, or excessive drug use. Can be taken long term and needs be taken for a prolonged period at least 4-12 weeks to be of most benefit In disease like hepatitis you just use it by itself sometimes for months after this time you can consider adding Dandelion.

Used to increase milk production in mothers and for gallbladder problems.

Uses - Liver problems, gallbladder problems, hepatitis, to increase milk production.

Dose - 1 tablespoon of seed given morning and night. Good for long term treatment.

Valerian

Actions - Sedative, antispasmodic, hypnotic, hypotensive, carminative.

A powerful nervine and sedative stronger than other herbal sedatives, pain reliever, reduces anxiety, hysteria, soothes the nervous system, reduces high blood pressure, slows and strengthens the heart and calms palpitations, useful for muscle spasms, arthritic pain, spinal injuries, aids indigestion and gas, insomnia, cramps, colic, can help with migraines. Valerian root is one of the most widely used herbal nervines for calming horses as it can relieve anxiety and excitability without reducing the horse's mental faculties or their physical ability to perform.

Uses - Treatment of epilepsy, hysteria, acute constipation, worms, malaria, pain and for sensitive nervous animals.

Externally - The oil is used as a rub for paralyzed limbs, cramps, swollen arteries and veins.

Dose - 1 to 2 tablespoons twice daily. Give more for a pain killing action.

Caution - Do not mix with drug tranquillizers.

Wild Yam

Actions - Antispasmodic, anti-inflammatory, anti-rheumatic,

The first birth control pills were once based on this remedy. Used for severe digestive pain in conditions such as colic, dysmenorrhea, and ovarian and uterine pains. Also used in the treatment of rheumatoid arthritis especially when there is painful inflammation. Muscle cramps and spasms, nerve pains and threatened miscarriage.

Dose - 1 tablespoon of powder twice daily.

Willow Bark (White Willow)

Actions - Febrifuge, bitter tonic, astringent, antiseptic, analgesic, anti-inflammatory, anti-rheumatic.

Willow Bark can be thought of as caveman's Aspirin as it was developed from this. Cattle and horses eat the young shoots and foliage. It is a refrigerant herb valuable in fevers and pain relief but can take a while to get into the system so think of looking for results especially in pain in about a day's time.

Uses - Treatment of all fevers, debility, enteritis, colic, pleurisy, rheumatism, sciatica and urinary infections as the excretion of salicylic acid in urine soothes a inflamed tract.

Externally - Rickets and cramp.

Dose - 2 teaspoonful's of powdered bark twice daily.

Externally - Use the same brew as a massage in pain

effected areas.

Wood Betony

Actions - Alterative, analgesic, antispasmodic, astringent, Bitter tonic, sedative, circulatory stimulant, diuretic.

Juliette de Bairacli Levy says the whole plant possesses a pungent and peculiar aroma especially when trampled on. This would show the plant to have a high oil content. Was once used as a smoke and snuff to treat headaches. Wood Betony is used for severe pains in the face and head consider it for horses with severe sinus or those who always toss there head.

Uses - Treatment of debility, gastritis, diarrhea, acidity, glandular deficiency, arthritis, rheumatism, exhaustion, sciatica, hypertension, kidney dysfunction.

Externally - arthritis, rheumatism, sciatica, rickets, tumors, swellings, boils, abscesses, corns, warts and blisters, gingivitis, as a poultice to draw out splinters and boils.

Dose - 2 handfuls made into a syrup by simmering in 1 and a half pints of water to which has been added a quarter pound of brown sugar or half a cup full of the dried herb twice daily.

Yellow Dock

Actions - Alterative, Cholagogue, purgative, mild

astringent.

A powerful blood purifier and astringent. It is used in treating all diseases of the blood and skin. Very high in iron, making it useful for treating anemia. It nourishes and detoxifies the liver and cleanses and enriches the blood.

Used extensively for skin complaints such as psoriasis, a mild acting remedy for the relief of constipation has an action on the gallbladder.

Uses - Constipation, skin problems, gallbladder problems, jaundice.

Dose - 1 tablespoon of powder twice daily, less if purgative action is to much.

Homeopathic Supplement

Homeopathy has been around now for hundreds of years and unlike most other forms of medicine its rules have not changed and will not for they are based on a essential truth. The main rule is Like cures Like or if we break down the word Homeopathy homo means the same and pathy means disease. As Homoeopathy is a very hard science to learn and as it kind of sits or balances on the border of hard science and metaphysics I will not try to explain to you what it is here as it would probably take a whole book to do this but I will say this, in the UK and a lot of countries in Europe it is on and paid for by the National Health System and anything that can get a politician to open their purse must work.

It is said that Homeopathy sits on a three legged stool. What this means is that if a remedy has at least three symptoms in the same strength as the symptoms you are trying to match then that remedy is a potential cure for your condition or if not cure it will offer the condition relief. The more symptoms you can match to the remedy the better the remedy will work for the rule is likes cure likes not vaguely similar cures. Listed below are some common Homoeopathic Remedies and some of the symptoms they cover. The idea is to find one remedy that covers most of your symptoms. To make the remedies as closer a match as we can we ask lots of questions like the ones below and after we gather all the answers we have what is called a good Symptom Picture which we then try to match as accurately as we can to a Remedy. Most Homeopathic Materia Medicas are set out to answer the questions listed below with the mind symptoms being the most important. Questions on time, position and temperature are good for making a choice between to very close remedies. The best Materia Medica for the lay person is Boerickes and you should be able to view this on a few Homeopathic websites.

Symptom Guide Questions

1. Was there a sudden onset of the condition, at what time?
2. What time of the day does the patient feel either better or worse.
3. What is the effect of motion? jarring? walking? running?
4. What is the effect of drinking fluids? warm and or cold drinks?
5. Is the patient thirsty or not at all? sips or gulps?
6. Is the onset from exertion? overeating? weather changes? emotions?
7. Mental emotional state of patient?
8. Better warm room? warm air?
9. Better cool room? cool open air?
10 Are the respirations upper chest movements or in the abdomen?
11 Respirations - dry or wet?

12 Expectoration - watery or stringy mucous, easy or difficult.

13 Is there coughing

14 Position - better or worse from sitting? standing? lying? lying on which side?

15 Along with the condition is there fever? gas? belching? wind?

Modality - The questions above are covering what the Homoeopaths call modalities which basically mean are covering a condition that makes the patient better or worse. I will list the main Modalities below. The Modalities help us to distinguish which remedy is right for the case especially when we have a group that look as though they may all work which is what I am giving you und the disease heading. Using modalities forces you to think what really is going on, is this the nature of the beast or the nature of the disease.

Time - Better or Worse morning, night, weekly, monthly, seasonally etc.

Motion - Better or Worse first movement, rest, exertion, walking, stretching, rising up etc

Temperature - Better or Worse heat, cold, cold air blowing, sudden change etc.

Body Activity - Better or Worse eating, drinking, urinating, defecating, sleep, coughing etc

Weather - - Better or Worse, damp, sunny, foggy, storms, sudden changes etc.

Senses - Better or Worse - touch, pressure, noise,

light, odors etc.

Position - Better or Worse lying, standing, sitting, stretched out, doubled up, right side etc.

Mind - Excitement, anger, fear, stress, better busy, nervous all the time etc.

Now read through all the remedies in the Marteria Medica (Homoeopathic Remedy Reference) and you will notice that most of them have Mind or mental symptoms kind of describing the personalities or moods a good example is Nux Vomica, I think we all know a nasty type of individual that this remedy would be suited to and meaning as though the individual is suited to this remedy then the remedy would have a curative action on them but don't expect it to change the nature of the beast. One of the main rules of Homeopathy is the closer the match of the remedy the higher the Potency you use but if you are not used to Homoeopathy just use the 30C potency and remember what I said about the 3 legged stool. Potency is a measure of strength and depth of action.

Remember as mentioned before Homoeopathy sits on a three legged stool. What this means is that if a remedy has at least three symptoms in the same strength as your symptoms then that remedy is a potential cure.

Note - The best prescribing guide for the layman is **Boerickes Materia Medica With Repertory.**

Another good guide is **The Complete Book Of Homeopathy by Dr Michael Weiner.**

I always buy my books on Homeopathy from India as they are quarter the price and there is always a wide selection. Put B. Jain Publishers into the google search engine go to their web site and check out these books and I am sure you will be pleased with what you find.

Disease Nosodes

Nosodes are remedies made from disease material mainly from the tissues, discharges, exudates, excretions, suppurations or secretions of a infected being. Simply stated a Nosode is a homeopathic remedy prepared from a pathological specimen. Rabies Nosode, for example starts with the saliva of a rabid dog and is then potentized.

Nosodes have many uses and are widely used in homeopathic practice to help limit cases of infectious diseases and to help during the recovery phase of a disease especially the ones that linger and drag on. There are Nosodes for most infectious diseases of animals and humans the use of Nosodes in this way is referred to as isopathy rather than Homoeopathy. They are often used in farm situations, to limit the spread and the effects of infectious diseases. This has especially been used as a vital component of mastitis control on many farms, both organic and conventional. One documented event about Nosodes dates back to Napoleon marching his Legions through Europe and spreading Typhoid in their wake, the towns that had the best cure rates were the ones where the local Homoeopaths used a Nosode of the disease.

Nosodes can be used in the prevention of infectious diseases in the manner of vaccination but they work by a completely different mechanism then from the raising of antibodies that vaccines work by. As yet it is not actually known how they work but they have survived hundreds of years ridicule by producing results and will carry on doing so.

The best known study into Nosodes was done by Dr. Christopher Day of England involving 'kennel cough' in a boarding kennel. At the time he was called in, there were 40 dogs in the kennel with 35 that had kennel cough. About half had been vaccinated for this malady. He gave a Nosode to all the animals that were there and all the dogs that came in through the rest of the summer, which was another 214 dogs. He successfully reduced the incidence of kennel cough from over 90% to less than 2%.

Nosodes used for the prevention of diseases are usually given in the 30C potency. A good dosing regime is one dose given night and morning for 3 days followed by one per month for the next 6 months. This generally provides a good level of protection after the first week. A good example of how this can be used is a puppy given the Nosode of Parvovirus at 3 to 4 weeks of age instead of having to wait for 9 weeks for the vaccination, this way the puppy is protected before given the vaccination.

Nosodes can have homeopathic therapeutic properties in their own right. Such Nosodes are found in the Homoeopathic Materia Medica and have undergone a proper 'proving'. Examples are Bacillinum, Carcinosinum, Medorrhinum, Psorinum, Tuberculinum.

Dose - Dr. Surjit S. Makker recommends 20ml of remedy mixed with 8 liters of water for 100 birds. This medicated water should be shaken well and put in drinkers accordingly. For individual birds give them 2-3 pellets by mouth and keep them calm.

Notes

Materia Medica

Note - All Homeopathic Remedies are given in Potency and not in material Form.

Aconite

Characteristics - Aconite is best used in the first stages of a illness, especially when fear and anxiety are present. Symptoms appear suddenly, without warning and they may be caused by exposure to cold winds or draughts or by a severe fright. Symptoms are a marked restlessness, animal displays extreme anxiety or fear, high fever with a burning skin, extreme sweating and a burning thirst, a hoarse dry painful cough, bright light noises stress and cold worsen the symptoms, rest and quiet relieves the symptoms. The pains of Aconite are unbearable, sharp, shooting, burning pains, tingling and numbness. A remedy for fevers and inflammatory states, use at the first sign of all fevers, shivering with cold sweats, difficult breathing, animal shows desire for large quantities of water, symptoms worse at midnight, symptoms improve in the open air.

Mind - Great fear, anxiety, restlessness, extreme sensitivity to pain, worry, foreboding.

Better - In open air, warmth, rest.

Worse - In the evening and night, particularly before midnight, lying on affected side.

Allium Cepa

Characteristics - Increased secretions from the eyes and nose, like those of the common cold. Frequent sneezing with watery discharge which burns the nose and upper lip, but the eye discharge is bland and doesn't burn (the opposite of Euphrasia). Tickling in the throat with incessant cough (feels as if larynx is split) holds throat when coughing. Being in cool open air relieves the symptoms, eyelids are swollen and red, abdominal tympany with wind, this remedy is indicated in the early stages of most catarrhal conditions, mild forms of cat flu can be cut short if given early.

Better - Cold room (except cough), open air.

Worse - Evening, warm room, odors.

Antimonium Tartaricum - Ant Tart

Characteristics - Is characterized by a loose rattling unproductive cough such as is often herd in cats. Respiration can be very difficult with much gasping. There is usually thirst for little and often. Symptoms are worse in the evening, lying down and in cold damp weather or a warm room. Confined largely to respiratory diseases, abundant bronchial secretions, great rattling of mucous with little expectoration, drowsiness, debility and sweat.

Mind - Drowsy and despondent, fear of being alone, child will not be touched without whining.

Better - Sitting erect, from burping and

expectoration.

Worse - Evenings, lying down, damp cold weather.

Apis

Characteristics - Apis is used for various types of swelling and inflammation such as that from animal bites and bites and stings from insects, it is also used for measles, mumps, sore throats, sore red eyes and fever. Apis is a quick acting remedy for inflammations especially those ones with edema and lots of swelling which is its main use. Acute nephritis with scanty and burning urine there may be some blood in the urine. . Symptoms are swelling with edema which makes the effected parts look shiny, red and puffy, the swollen parts feel soggy and waterlogged, a fever that develops rapidly but without thirst, extreme restlessness and fidgeting, an irritable nature and perhaps jealous, cool air and cold compresses relieve the symptoms. Pains are burning and stinging, arthritis with swelling, animals seek cold surface to lie on, swollen eyelids, may be swollen ears, may be blood in the urine, in the horse and cow there may be edema in the lower limbs while in dogs abdominal dropsy is seen. Symptoms get worse from heat and improve in the open air and from cold bathing.

Mind - Apathy, indifference, awkward.

Better - By cold, (room, air or application)

Worse - From warmth, pressure, late in the

afternoon, from sleeping.

Arnica

Characteristics - Bruises and similar injuries where the skin is unbroken and there is mental or emotional shock. Symptoms are any type of bruising or similar injury caused by crushing, squeezing or wrenching, muscles strains which feel sore and bruised, shock after accidents, there is a fear of being touched because of the pain, good for the soreness after birth and medical operations.

Arnica can be used in potency and also as a cream. The cream must not be used on broken skin or wounds. Animal shrinks away when you try to touch it, symptoms improve when lying down.

Mind - Fears touch or approach, whole body oversensitive.

Better - Lying down or with head low.

Worse - Least touch, motion, damp and cold.

Arsenic Album

Characteristics - Burning pains relieved by heat, anxious, restless, weak and chilly with an air of fear and hopelessness. Anxiety or restlessness are often present where this remedy is indicated. Discharge from eyes and nose are watery and acrid causing ulceration in those regions. The mouth is usually dry and the patient is usually thirsty. Dramatic vomiting and diarrhea often simultaneously indicate its use if the modalities agree. The patient may have wheezing respiration and allergic asthmatic conditions can respond well. The skin can be dry, scaly and scruffy. Symptoms are worse for cold and wet better for warmth. Tries to find relief in motion but immediately feels weak with movement. Restless, feels cold, complains of general weakness, discharges burn the skin.

Mind - Fear with despair and restlessness.

Better - Warmth, open air, relieved by sweat, hot drinks, lying down (but restless).

Worse - Cold air, after midnight eg 1 to 3am. Wet damp weather and near sea shore.

Belladonna

Characteristics - This is one of the great fever remedies, conditions requiring its use usually being of violent and sudden onset. Heat, redness, pain and swelling characterize its symptoms. It is one of the main remedies used in convulsions. Pupils are usually dilated which is a keynote for this remedy. Acute ear inflammation where there is heat, pain and swelling respond well. The mouth is usually dry and there is great thirst. With Belladonna always think BIRDS. B for burning, I for irritability, R for redness, D for delirium and S for spasms.

Mind - Hallucinations, delirium, rages, bites, strikes, desire to escape.

Better - For quiet, dark, rest with slight warmth.

Worse - For noise, touch or jarring motion.

Bellis Perennis

Characteristics - Trauma to abdomen and pelvic organs especially after surgery and child birth if arnica does not give relief. Injuries to the nerves with intense soreness, back ache from hard physical work such as gardening, pain is bruised sore and aching, better cold presses, worse touch, after getting wet.

The animal is unwilling to move and when made to do so evinces pain, muscular stiffness is prominent.

Worse - Left side and cold wind.

Bryonia

Characteristics - This remedy shows both diarrhea and constipation symptoms, the latter usually in chronic conditions. The mouth is often dry and there is great thirst. The tongue is often coated yellow. It is of great help in many cases of rheumatism or arthritis where the symptoms agree. There is often respiratory signs with a hoarse hacking cough. All symptoms are worse for movement and better for rest.

Mind - Irritable, delirium.

Better - Lying on the painful side, pressure, rest and cold things.

Worse - Warmth, motion, morning, eating and touch.

Calendula

Characteristics - The part used is the Flowers and it is used for wounds and skin irritations, it is healing, soothing, anti-inflammatory, astringent, anti-fungal and anti-microbial.

Use as a lotion for cuts, grazes, infected sores, fungal infections, any skin inflammations, regulates the oil production of the skin so is good for acne, to stop bleeding, for bruises and sprains, skin ulcers and minor burns and scolds.

Note - The tincture of this is used as a lotion diluted at 1 to 10.

Cantharis

Characteristics - Important first aid remedy for minor burns and for other pains that feel burning and fiery, also has a healing effect on the bladder, urethra and other parts of the urinary tract where burning pain is the key symptom, burns and scalds especially where blistering and inflammation occur, sunburn, insect bites that feel hot and burn, cystitis. Pains are violent burning, cutting, stabbing or smarting, rawness, use when the animal appears distressed when passing urine, or tries to pass and cannot. Better from warmth rest and rubbing.

Mind - Furious delirium, acute mania generally of a sexual type, crying, barking.

Better - From rubbing

Worse - From touch or approach, from urinating,

from drinking cold water.

Carbo Vegetabilis

Characteristics - Patient exhibits mental and physical sluggishness and symptoms come on slowly, generalized weakness of all functions especially digestion, overweight, torpid, lazy, complaints of coldness, pains usually described as burning, pressing pains, wishes to be fanned, digestive problems such as belching often accompany any illness.

Mind - Aversion to darkness, sudden loss of memory.

Better - Being fanned, passing gas, rest.

Worse - Morning and evening, exertion, cold, tight clothes at abdomen.

Causticum

Characteristics - Burns and burning pains such as cystitis also used for dry coughs, burns to the skin especially with marked inflammation and blistering, coughs, laryngitis and hoarseness from straining and over using voice, cystitis especially with involuntary passing of urine when coughing, chronic cystitis, exposure to cold dry air may make symptoms worse.

Mind - Least thing makes it cry, sad, hopeless. Ailments from long lasting grief.

Better - In damp wet weather, warmth.

Worse - Cold winds.

Euphrasia

Characteristics - Affects the mucous membranes of the eyes, nose and chest producing copious watery secretions,eye secretions cause smarting of the skin while the nose discharge is bland. Used for conjunctivitis, eye strain generally but especially from computers, eyes that feel sore and inflamed and look red, hay fever symptoms including a tickly throat, sneezing, a runny nose, and itchy red watering eyes. Sunlight wind and warmth worsen the symptoms. Use for Dogs who have had their head out of the window for to long, symptoms better in dim light or darkness, in all species a tendency to diarrhea occurs.

Better - In the dark

Worse - From light, indoors, in the evening.

Hypericum

Characteristics - Used for bruises and other injuries especially to nerve rich areas like the fingers, lips, ears, eyes ,tail bone, good for the pain of puncture wounds of any cause eg animal or insect. Helps with the pains after operations especially amputations. Pains are violent shooting pains along a nerve path, burning, tingling and numbness. Worse from shock and touch and better from rubbing, horse fly bites, symptoms worse cold better warmth.

Mind - Anxiety, melancholy, effects of shock.

Better - Bending head backward.

Worse - Cold, dampness and touch.

Ipecac

Characteristics - Indicated for complaints of persistent nausea not relieved by vomiting, ailments caused by eating rich or indigestible type of foods such as ice-cream, sweets etc., useful to stop bleeding if blood is bright red.

Mind - Easily irritated, child cries or screams continuously, wanting something but not sure what they desire, holds everything in contempt.

Worse - Warm, moist weather, lying down.

Kali Bichromicum

Characteristics - Has a affinity for the mucous membranes of the body, tough stringy viscid secretions sometimes forming thick yellow green mucous, sinus infections, suited for fleshy fat light complexioned people, general weakness.

Better - Heat

Worse - Cold, beer, morning, undressing.

Kali Carbonicum

Characteristics - Has a affinity for the mucous membranes digestive and respiratory, very tired, anemic, flabby tissues which may be swollen, sweat, backache, weakness, many conditions have a aggravation at 2am to 4am, often stays immobile when ill.

Mind - Very irritable, hypersensitive to pain, despondent.

Better - During the day, sitting down, bending forward, warmth.

Worse - Cold weather, between 2am and 4am.

Lachesis

Characteristics - Many symptoms tend to be left sided, cannot bear tight clothing, symptoms worse on awakening, symptoms relieved with onset of the menstrual flow. Short dry cough, feels relief after coughing up watery phlegm, feeling of constriction in throat and chest, better bending forward.

Mind - Overly talkative, impatient, sad, jealous, no desire to mix with world.

Better - Release of pressure, eating fruit, cold, discharges.

Worse - Pressure, touch, after sleep, heat, hot weather.

Ledum

Characteristics - Has a action on the capillaries and is useful for cleaning up bruises especially around the eyes, mainly used for puncture wounds made by sharp points such as nails and wood splinters and insect bites and stings especially ones that don't heal properly and look blue and puffy. Wounds that feel cold to the touch, septic conditions, sprains, pains are throbbing, tearing ,prickling, they shoot upwards, stiff and sore. Better cold, cold bathing. This remedy was used in the past along with hypericum to ward off tetanus especially in deep wounds

Better - From cold.

Worse - At night and from heat.

Lycopodium

Characteristics - Exerts most of its effects on the digestive organs, liver, kidneys and respiratory systems. The patient dislikes being left alone and appears apprehensive. The nose is often blocked and there may be blisters on the tongue. Eating a little food always satisfies the appetite but appetite is very marked. The belly is usually bloated. The stool appears hard and small and is expelled only with difficulty accompanied by ineffectual straining. Urination is also a slow process and the urine has a red sediment. Symptoms are worse for heat generally and better for cold.

Mind - Melancholy, afraid to be alone, apprehensive.

Better - By motion, on getting cold.

Worse - From heat.

Natrum Sulphuricum

Characteristics - A good liver remedy, emotional and mental difficulties arising after head injury, useful in problems associated with rainy weather and dampness, patient feels every change from dry to wet weather, may remove excess water and fluid retention from the body.

Mind - Lively music saddens, melancholy, inability to think, dislikes to speak or be spoken to.

Better - Dry weather and environments, pressure, change of position.

Worse - Damp weather, damp basements, lying on left side.

Nux Vom

Characteristics - The remedy for overindulgence, adapted especially to thin irritable energetic people who attend with great detail to tasks, quarrelsome, nervous, intelligent, hypochondriacal, oversensitive to noise music and light, craves stimulants.

Primarily used in the digestive sphere, its greatest reputation is in helping disturbances following overeating of unsuitable foods. Feces is usually hard but diarrhea can follow overeating. There is abdominal discomfort, flatulence, irritability and sensitivity to noise. Symptoms are generally worse for noise and better after rest or for damp weather.

Mind - Very irritable, sensitive to all impressions, malicious, disposed to reproach others.

Better - Wet weather, lying down, uninterrupted nap.

Worse - Overeating, mental over exertion, sensory stimulation ie sound, sight, touch etc.

Phosphorus

Characteristics - Irritated and inflamed mucous and serous membranes are the key feature of this remedy. Is a very sudden remedy with suddenness of symptoms. The patient is sensitive to loud and sudden noises (eg thunder fireworks etc). Degenerative processes and bone destruction respond well to Phosphorus. Food is suddenly vomited back up when it has been warmed in the stomach, gums can be ulcerated and bloody. Hepatitis, jaundice, pancreatic disease and nephritis come into its sphere. Urine may be bloody. A very painful cough is also a symptom. Wounds that perpetually bleed may also be helped. The patient is usually in poor body condition. Symptoms are worse for touch, exertion, in the evening and during thunder storm. Better for cold and sleep.

Mind - Low spirits, restless, fidgety.

Better - In the dark, lying on the right side, from the cold, sleep.

Worse - Touch, from exertion and in the evening.

Pulsatilla

Characteristics - Often indicated for those with mild, gentle, timid yielding dispositions who are easily moved to laughter and tears, The Pulsatilla person wants to be held and loved, moods changeable and fickle, the patient is chilly but desires strolling in cold air, symptoms are erratic and change frequently, pains are wandering, pains that grow gradually in intensity, fever without thirst despite dry mouth, bland yellow discharges.

Mind - Weeps easily, timid, fears to be alone - dark - ghosts, likes sympathy and fuss, highly emotional, easily discouraged, sensitive.

Better - Open air, cold applications, consolation relieves symptoms.

Worse - Evening before midnight, warmth, after eating fat rich food.

Rhus Tox

Characteristics - Is the most famous of the rheumatic remedies. The skin and muscular skeletal system are its main spheres. Small red papules in the skin and sometimes vesicles are typical lesions with much scratching. In all cases of damage to muscles think of Rhus and the symptoms of arthritis which are worse after rest particularly if this follows strenuous exertion. The symptoms improve with limbering up , The worst pains are seen as the animal arises from its bed.

Mind - Listless, sad, extreme restlessness, great apprehension at night.

Better - Warmth, walking, from stretching out limbs.

Worse - During sleep, cold wet rainy weather and at night.

Ruta

Characteristics - Has effects on the joints, tendons, cartilages, and the periosteum which is a fine membrane that covers bones and gives it that shiny look, it is also used for eye strain where the vision goes dim.

Used for painful bruises affecting the bones, dislocations, strains to the tendons or joints, aching with restlessness, pains are gnawing, digging, burning, bruised, sore as if beaten, bones as if broken, pain deep in the bones, rheumatism.

Better - From lying and warmth.

Worse - From over exertion, touch, cold wet weather.

Silica

Characteristics - Fits the shy chilly patient who is reluctant to enter the room, chronic inflammatory conditions such as sinus, helps in the removal of foreign bodies such as splinters and seeds, ripens abscesses, ailments attended with pus formation. Use silica and be prepared to use it for a while sometimes up to 3 weeks.

Mind - Faint hearted, anxious, yielding.

Better - Warmth, wet or humid weather.

Worse - Morning, from lying down, cold.

Staphysagria

Characteristics - Suits sensitive people who suppress their feelings and suffer in silence or who boil over with indignation, remedy for cuts and wounds especially those that are from medical procedures and have the mentioned feelings. Nervous states of animals. The pains are stinging, stitching, smarting, squeezing, as if stabbed by a knife. Worse from touch, emotions and suppressed anger.

Better - Warmth, rest at night.

Worse - Touch on affected parts, loss of fluids.

Symphytum

Characteristics - Causes bone to grow and promotes fast healing should be given for all fractures. Used for injuries to the hard parts of the body while arnica is for the soft parts. Also used for eye injuries caused from blows.

Caution - do not use if a pin has been placed in the bone as the pin has to be removed latter.

Tarentula Cubensis

Characteristics - For abscesses, boils, carbuncles, swellings of any kind but especially on the back of the neck where the skin turns black, red/blue or purple with great pain. Deep septic conditions with hardening of the effected part, condition comes on fast, pains are burning, stinging, throbbing, pricking like a needle.

Worse - Night.

Urtica Urens

Characteristics - Can be used for burns and also for cystitis where the urine burns the skin and there is dificulty passing urine. Symptoms are stinging pains, swellings particularly blistery swellings, itching.

Worse - Cool moist air, touch.

Notes

Vitamin C

Vitamin C is the primary antioxidant in the lungs and a powerful antihistamine without side effects. Low vitamin C dramatically increases histamine levels which put you at greater risks for inflammation responses in the body. Always give a high dose of Vitamin C to animals before any operation where they require a anesthetic for the reasons mentioned above as they will recover faster and better from the anesthetic and maybe the inflammation from the surgical incisions will be toned down a bit.

Vitamin C is needed by the immune system and is necessary for healing and the prevention of infections along with being a potent antioxidant with anti-bacterial and antiviral actions. It is also essential for the utilization of the essential amino acids lysine (anti-viral) and proline. Another point to consider is that stress depletes the bodies supply of Vitamin C so this may be another factor in the cause of many diseases. Vit C is essential for the formation of collagen tissue which is vital in tendons and cartilage so always consider this in muscle and back injuries and especially trauma injuries.

Sodium Ascorbate is good for use on animals as it is virtually tasteless when added to the animal's food and does not curdle milk. This can be used in high doses when needed for example dose till the bowels become loose then back the dose off. For severe situations you can use a injectable Vitamin C, in Australia we use Troys Injectable Vit C which we get from the Agricultural Stock Feed Shops or Co Ops. Use a large gauge needle with this as some animals have rather thick hides and the liquid solution is also fairly thick.

Think of using Vitamin C in all operations and all acute diseases. It is a good last resort to think of before the rifle especially in the deadly acute diseases where as a last resort you would use the injectable form in a intramuscular injection, this can also be a good gauge as to what may happen as these injections hurt like hell so if the animal turns around and gives you a filthy look then there is a good chance that they may live and if they do not seem to notice the injection well the chances don't look too good. So remember always keep a bottle of Injectable C in the fridge for emergencies.

Good Herb Sources Of Vitamin C

Alfalfa, Burdock, Catnip, Cayenne, Chickweed, Dandelion, Hawthorn, Garlic, Horseradish, Kelp, Parsley, Plantain, Papaya, Raspberry, Rosehips, Shepherds Purse, Yellow Dock.

The Safest Essential Oils For Animal Use

Supplement To The Natural Remedies For Animal Series

Extreme care must be taken using the Essential Oils on animals. The ones mentioned in these pages seem to be the safest if used in a low dose which is a quarter of what you would use on a human and even this would be too high if used on a mouse so really think about what you are doing and always use a little test dose to check for sensitivity.

Danger - Do not use on **birds** and **cats** as there metabolism cannot handle Essential oils and death will be the most likely result, this includes Eucalyptus and Tea Tree oil.

How Oils Work

Essential Oils work by entering the blood stream via the pores of the skin so the biggest action is on the area applied followed by a systemic action via the blood. The liver is the main blood filter and detoxifier of the body so the liver is responsible for breaking down any drug or blood borne foreigner so with the Essential Oils there is always the chance that if the dose is too high or the application is to frequent the liver may be damaged. Never forget that oils are highly concentrated products. A good example is a budgie, you clipped the wings and one is now bleeding so you put Tea Tree oil on it. Imagine the size of one drop of oil now imagine the size of a Budgies liver and it's fairly obvious what's going to happen.

Below are given the cautions for using oils on dogs, follow these cautions on all animals in general. Most information for these pages was sourced from Kristen Leigh Bells book Holistic Aromatherapy For Animals and Catharine Birds book A Healthy Horse The Natural Way.

Essential Oil Blends

Soothing Skin Essential Oil Blend

15ml base oil of hazel nut or sweet almond oil

2 drops Geranium

6 drops Rosewood

6 drops Lavender

1 drop Roman Chamomile

2 drops Carrot Seed

Combine all ingredients, shake and store in a dark glass bottle. Use 2 to 4 drops of this blend to spot treat small areas of skin.

Mange Treatment Blend

15ml base oil of hazel nut or sweet almond oil

5 drops Lavender

7 drops Niaouli

1 drop Helichrysum

2 drops Sweet Marjoram

After bathing the dog 2 to 4 drops of the blend should be applied to the affected areas twice a day for at least 2 weeks. Observe for a week and repeat if necessary. Try to prevent the dog from licking the area.

Tick Bite Forula
15ml base oil of hazel nut or sweet almond oil
5 drops Thyme Thujanol
3 drops Hyssop Decumbens
8 drops Lavender
For use on bites or immediately after the tick is removed to help prevent infection, reduce redness and inflammation and possibly prevent Lymes disease.

Fresh Breath Oil Blend
5ml base oil of hazel nut or sweet almond oil
6 drops Cardamom
4 drops Coriander Seed
6 drops Peppermint
1 to 3 drops inside of the dogs mouth.

Calm Dog Blend
15ml base oil of hazel nut or sweet almond oil
3 drops Valerian
2 drops Vetiver
4 drops Petitgrain
3 drops Sweet Marjoram
2 drops Sweet Orange
The calming effect ranges from taking the edge off to soothing the dog. Dose is 1 to 6 drops depending on the size of the dog.

Fear or Seperation Anxiety

15ml base oil of hazel nut or sweet almond oil
1 drop Neroli
2 drops Sweet Bazil
4 drops Bergamot
6 drops Petitgrain
1 drop Ylang Ylang
Dose is 1 to 6 drops depending on size of dog.

Flea Free Blend

15ml base oil of hazel nut or sweet almond oil
4 drops Clary Sage
1 drop Citronella
7 drops Peppermint
3 drops Lemon
Store in dark glass bottle. 2 to 4 drops to the neck, chest, legs and tail base of the dog.

Tick Free Blend

15ml base oil of hazel nut or sweet almond oil
2 drops Geranium
2 drops Rosewood
3 drops Lavender
2 drops Myrhh
2 drops Opoponax
1 drop Bay Leaf
Store in dark glass bottle. 2 to 4 drops to the neck, chest, legs and tail base of the dog.

Increasing The Appetite

15ml base oil of hazel nut or sweet almond oil

2 drops Sweet Orange

2 drops Lemon

2 drops Grapefruit

2 drops Lime

2 drops Bergamot

For old and sick dogs this is a gentle appetite stimulant. 2 to 6 drops of the final blend to the neck and chest of the dog gently rubbed in. Repeat as needed up to 6 times per day.

Immune Boosting Blend

15ml base oil of hazel nut or sweet almond oil

2 drops Bay Laurel

2 drops Ravensare

2 drops Palmarosa

2 drops Eucalyptus

2 drops Niaouli

2 drops Coriander Seed

2 drops Thyme Thujanol

2 to 4 drops daily via massage to neck and chest.

Colds and Congestion

15ml base oil of hazel nut or sweet almond oil

5 drops Eucalyptus

5 drops Myrhh

5 drops Ravensare

For relieving nasal congestion or cold symptoms in dogs. 1 to 6 drops rubbed into neck or chest.

Fatigue Blend

15ml base oil of hazel nut or sweet almond oil

7 drops Rosemary

6 drops Tangerine

3 drops Ylang Ylang

Balancing and revitalizing for dogs that are suffering from fatigue and malaise.

2 to 4 drops daily via massage to neck and chest.

Flatulence Blend

15ml base oil of hazel nut or sweet almond oil

3 drops Caraway

3 drops Cardamom

3 drops Cinnamon

3 drops Nutmeg

3 drops Tangerine

1 to 2 drops placed on your dog's food and then 1 or 2 drops given after eating. Many dogs enjoy the taste of this spicy blend and will lick it off your hand. The spice oils of this blend are commonly found in food flavorings so digestion is regarded as safe.

Joint Rub Blend

15ml base oil of hazel nut or sweet almond oil

3 drops Black Pepper

4 drops Peppermint

3 drops Speramint

4 drops Juniper Berry

Good for muscle soreness, arthritis, hip dysplasia and sprains. use 2 to 4 drops of the blend and try to rub in as close to the skin as possible. Do a patch test with this oil as it can be irritating. Patch tests can be done with drop of blend in the arm pit.

Motion Sickness Blend
15ml base oil of hazel nut or sweet almond oil
7 drops Ginger
8 drops Peppermint
Give 3 drops in the mouth

Labor Ease Blend
15ml base oil of hazel nut or sweet almond oil
6 drops Clary Sage
1 drop Neroli
5 drops Petitgrain
2 drops Lavender
1 drop Roman Chamomile
Calming and balancing blend, can be applied to the fur of the neck or chest or 1 to 4 drops can be rubbed in the belly.

Oils For Horses

The safest way to use Essential Oils on your horse are external massage and inhalation. When inhaled the Oil addresses the horses emotional states and stored memories as well as entering the body and having an effect with the most obvious here being Eucalyptus which acts as a bronchodilator (illegal for competition horses in some parts of the US). **Use blends in the same strengths as mentioned in dogs don't go over 2% oil in a blend. Only apply the** blends to the affected areas. You can copy some of the dog formulas or make your own using the list of oils.

Essential Oils For Animal Use

The Essential Oils below are fairly safe for Animal Use

Basil (Sweet) - Helpful for restoring mental balance and clarity. For animals that are suffering nervousness or anxiety, dogs with separation anxiety. Use sparingly (PMC30%). **Horses** - Helps to release most muscle spasms. Used before a event it minimizes the amount of uric acid in the blood and other toxic wastes from exercise. A warming winter oil feeding the muscle fibers and stimulating the blood flow. It is a expectorant removing mucous from a clogged respiratory system when rubbed into the chest and inhaled. Rubbed into the abdomen it may help to relieve the pain and symptoms of colic. May irritate the skin in high doses and don't use in pregnancy.

Bay Leaf - Good for a hair and fur tonic, ticks don't like it, good deodorizer.

Actions - Ant microbial.

Bay Laurel - Used in blends for boosting the immune system especially in dogs. Use only in small amounts in blends.

Bergamot - Combines toning, strengthening and balancing effects with soothing, relaxing and uplifting qualities. Useful for the treatment of fungal conditions such as dog ear infections due to yeast overgrowth. Use in small doses as it can cause photosensitization. **Horse** - Use full for treating any skin complaint especially folliculitis, flaking skin and wounds. Good for lice infections and bites, aids in the healing of any wounds and reduces scar formation. Has a stimulating effect on appetite. Be cautious when applying to the skin of a gray horse or to sensitive skin areas that will be exposed to the sun as this oil can cause photosensitization or pigment changes.

Black Pepper - Warming and circulatory stimulant qualities with low toxicity and irritation. Good for sore muscles, joint pains, arthritis and hip dysplasia. **Horse** - Gives tone to skeletal muscles and warms any winter chills. Dilates local blood vessels and improves local blood flow to the muscles warming the muscles from inside. Arthritic joints respond well to pepper and helps with pain management when used over a long period of time. Strengthens the nervous system. May antidote Homoeopathics.

Caraway Seed - Good for digestive problems, wind, poor appetite, indigestion and bad breath.

Cardamom - Digestive problems, bad breath. **Horse** - Good for treating digestive problems of a nervous origin. Encourages the flow of saliva and good for loss of appetite. It is warming when the body feels cold and useful for easing coughs and respiratory complaints. Highly antiviral and second only to

Eucalyptus in that respect. For stallions you can use it as an aphrodisiac. May irritate some sensitive skins.

Carrot Seed - Valuable oil in the use of skin care, dry flaky skin that is sensitive to allergens and prone to infections. **Horses** - Strengthens the mucous membranes so is good for respiratory conditions. Useful for regenerating the skin after wounds or skin diseases and it antiseptic action will deal with minor infections. Has a toning hormone like action that will encourage conception and assist the infertile mare.

Cedarwood Atlas - Gentle stimulating oil that increases circulation and stimulates the release toxins. Good for the skin and fleas don't like it. **Horse** - Sores that are slow to heal, saddle sores, folliculitis etc. and dry flaky skin, encourage the re-growth of coat and adds shine. Has a tonic effect on the kidneys. Dries out excess phlegm and runny noses and removes excess mucous from the respiratory system when inhaled.

Chamomile German - Powerful skin soothing ant inflammatory. Burns, allergic reaction and all types of skin irritations can be quickly calmed with this oil. The oil has a deep blue color.

Chamomile Roman - Valuable for soothing the central nervous system and relieving cramps spasms and muscle pains. It also has analgesic effects which may be used for wounds. In humans this has traditionally been used for teething. **Horse** - The strong analgesic properties relieve dull muscular aches and stubborn spasms. It can also relieve overworked and inflamed muscles. Can be used as a wash to relieve the pain of inflames wounds. Good for calming difficult and unruly horses. Good for unmanageable mares when they cycle.

Cinnamon Leaf - Use the leaf not the bark as the leaf is gentler. Excellent digestive tonic and good for flatulent dogs and is a powerful anti-microbial.

Citronella - Well known insect repeller.

Clary Sage - Sedates the central nervous system, good for calming blends. **Horse** - Has a strong regenerative power where hair loss is involved. Useful on puffy joints caused by long periods of standing. Any swelling in the kidney area caused by strenuous work or sluggish kidney function. Calms underlying tension and soothes anxiety. Useful for a mare having trouble conceiving or nervous of the stallion. Don't use during pregnancy.

Coriander Seed - A toning balancing and strengthening oil that promotes and supports the digestion. It is also a circulatory stimulant and thus a good addition to blends for sore joints, muscles or arthritis.

Eucalyptus Radiata - A well-known remedy for congestion of the respiratory system. The oil has anti-viral, anti-inflammatory and expectorant effects. Can be a flea repellant. Antidotes Homoeopathic remedies. **Horse** - Eases muscular aches and pains caused by over exertion, relieves rheumatic and nerve pains. The anti-viral action is good for respiratory infections and it also soothes the inflammation and reduces excess mucous. Heals sores prone to pus formation. Can be irritating to sensitive skin.

Frankincense - Used to strengthen a weakened immune system and is a good choice for any blend for a sick or elderly animal that needs a systemic boost. Can be used for skin aliments due to its anti-inflammatory and anti-bacterial qualities. Horse - Eases shortness of breath and helps any respiratory problem. Rejuvenating especially for those recovering from a serious injury, tonic for the aging and can be used as a pick me up. Good for stubborn hard to heal wounds. Has the ability to dispel fear and anxiety. Don't use during pregnancy.

Geranium - Has tonic and strong anti-fungal actions, suitable in the use of prevention and treatment of fungal ear infections. Also can be used in tick repellant formulas. **Horse** - Gentle analgesic, has diuretic properties and a tonic action on the liver and kidneys. Balance hormones and emotions so is good for erratic mood swings.

Ginger - Good for the digestive and circulatory systems. Used for motion sickness, sprains, strains and arthritis. **Horse** - Good for conditions caused by cold and dampness. Stimulates circulation to cold joints and is analgesic relieving arthritic and rheumatic pain, muscle spasms and sprains. Is a appetite stimulant and can relieve travel sickness. Careful on sensitive skins.

Grapefruit - Used for calming, deodorizing and also repelling insects particularly fleas. Has a tonic effect on skin, hair and tissues. Useful for animals with imbalanced sebum production. **Horse** - Gentle effective lymphatic stimulant that nourishes cells while removing toxins. Tonic to the liver. Careful on sensitive skins.

Helichrysum - Actions - Analgesic, anti-inflammatory, regenerative, good for the skin.

Hyssop Decumbens - Different from the normal hyssop. This one is a antiviral and antibacterial and anti-depressant. The oil is also nontoxic and irritating.

Juniper Berry - Stimulating to the circulatory system and good for use in blends used for arthritis and pain. Helpful for balancing oily skin and for acne, eczema and hair loss. **Horse** - Helps stimulate kidney function and this in turn helps to remove metabolic wastes. Don't use during pregnancy.

Labdunum - This oil is antibacterial and astringent. Used for wounds.

Lavender - Antibacterial, antipruritic (anti-itch), powerful regenerative properties. The oil acts as a sedative on the central nervous system. **Horse** - Is cell regenerating and hastens the healing process. Sedates and soothes any wound or emotion. Helps to dispel gas and eases muscle tightness.

Lemon - Calming, strong antibacterial, deodorizer. **Horse** - Stimulates the body to excrete toxins and wastes via the skin, gently astringent and encourages the movement and release of excess toxins. Supports the liver and kidneys. In the cold season gently addresses runny watery respiratory problems and boosts the immune system. For older horses it can be added to rheumatic blends.

Lemon Grass - Antiviral and has a calming effect. **Horse** - Relieves pain in aching muscles and makes the muscles supple. Careful on sensitive skin and around wounds.

Mandarin Green - Good for calming fear, anxiety or stress. **Horse** - Nourishes the peripheral circulation feeding any extremity that suffers from poor circulation. Helps with muscle spasms.

Marjoram - Calming, spasmolytic, strong antibacterial, bacterial infections, wound care and insect repelling.
Meant to be good for calming over amorous male dogs. **Horse** - Warms cold aching joints, relieves muscle spasms and draws bruising to the surface. Helps with the aches and pain of arthritis and swollen joints in old horses. Can help with travel sickness.

Myrrh - Anti-inflammatory, anti-viral, good for puppy teething, treating irritated or inflamed skin conditions or for adding to immune boosting blends. Good for repelling ticks. **Horse** - Its antiseptic action is useful for deep seated respiratory conditions when inhaled. Can be used in a compress to treat boils, chapped or weeping skin conditions and fungal conditions like ringworm. Has a stimulating toning action on the mares reproductive system. Use only short term and not during pregnancy.

Neroli - Calming, stress reduction, anxiety, used for blend for female dogs in labor to ease pain and stress.

Niaouli - Anti histamine, antibacterial, good for allergies manifesting on the skin as well as first aid. Use for cleaning and for preventing ear infections in dogs.

Nutmeg - Canine flatulence, reduces gas production and aids in indigestion and nausea. Stimulating to the circulatory system.

Sweet Orange - Calming, deodorizing, flea repellant, may help in excess sebum production of the skin.

Palmarosa - Antibacterial, antiviral. **Horse** - Helpful when the body is over heated, encourages cellular regeneration and aid hydration by encouraging the flow of fluids throughout the body. Good for stiff joints and aching back.

Patchouli - Gentle circulatory stimulant for the skin and coat and also acts as a insect repellant. **Horse** - Tissue regenerator that aids in the healing of wounds, may address old scar tissue if applied regularly. Used for treating sores that contain heat a compress will cool the wound and help heal. Helps the skin regain its elasticity. Has diuretic properties.

Peppermint - Stimulates circulation, analgesic, sprains, strains, arthritis, repels fleas, flies, mossies', itching, car sickness. **Horse** - Peppermint has a cooling and analgesic action on heated local injuries. Can burn sensitive skins. Antidotes Homoeopathics.

Ravensare - Anti viral and antibacterial. For animals with compromised immune systems or for young dogs that are prone to infections.

Rose - Stabilizing to the central nervous system, has a gentle tonifying effect to the skin good for adding to blends for itchy or irritated skin.

Rosemary - The oil is mucolytic acting as a expectorant and also aids in cell regeneration. May help in promoting and maintaining hair growth. **Horse** - Stimulates both the mental and physical body into action, can relieve pain without sedating.

Rosewood - The oil has antiviral and antibacterial properties and ticks are repelled by the scent of it. Good for skin conditions.

Spearmint - Similar actions to peppermint, repels fleas and other insects stimulates circulation to the area it is used.

Spikenarde - Calming and grounding, rejuvenating and regenerating to the skin, good for dogs with skin problems, has a similar range of action as valerian.

Thyme Linalol - Antibacterial, anti-fungal, good for skin problems and not as harsh as thyme.

Thyme Thujanol - Has all the benefits of the above thyme as well as being a immune system stimulant and live detoxifier. Can be used in the prevention of lymes disease applied immediately after a tick bite.

Valerian - Calming and grounding, good for dogs with separation anxiety or who are fearful of loud noises, storms, fireworks or new situations. Good as a tonic for the nervous system.

Vetiver - Used in blends for calming, circulatory

tonic and strengthens the immune system. **Horse -** Used to treat aches and pains and is a tonic for most body systems. Used for debilitated and distressed horses.

Ylang Ylang - Deeply calming, used in fatigue blends. **Horses** - Commonly used as a aphrodisiac, has an affinity for the adrenal glands.

Notes

Notes

Notes

Notes

Notes

Notes

www.ingramcontent.com/pod-product-compliance
Lightning Source LLC
Chambersburg PA
CBHW071406170526
45165CB00001B/194

* 9 7 8 1 4 8 2 5 0 6 5 9 4 *